This book is the j ____ T0161184 ____ the body works and how physical ailments ____ ___ __ ____ ___ ___ ___ ___ .1. Then it shows specific action steps that will allow the body to heal itself. I recommend this book to anyone interested in a healthy life.

—Bill Ferguson
Author and creator of *Mastery of Life*

As an allopathic medical doctor trained in Physical Medicine and Rehabilitation, I have been trained in working with a team of clinicians to optimize the functional recovery of patients who have become disabled due to injury or illnesses. More recently, I have completed a fellowship in Integrative Medicine, and my eyes have been opened to the benefits of holistic modalities addressing the mind-body-spirit connection. Your Body is a Self-Healing Machine Trilogy *is a perfect guide to those who want to partake in self-care and be co-creators of health and wellness. Especially in the current times, we live where we are constantly challenged to maintain our health, and this information is needed to reverse the damage we have done to our bodies and our environment.*

Understanding why our current health system is not working and why more people are getting sicker as our cost gets exponentially out of control is crucial to becoming empowered to initiate a change. This book gives us an excellent introduction to applied epigenetics and how we can use it to support our self-healing machine that can rebuild itself. Included are practical recommendations on making the optimal nutritional choices, detoxification, lifestyle choices, and addressing the emotional, mental, and spiritual body.

Our bodies need support for healing, but what is often not discussed is what we can do to prevent illness development in the first place. Understanding applied epigenetics will allow each of us to be proactive in our self-care and be part of the solution to our burgeoning healthcare crises. This book will be an excellent resource for my patients and those who want to improve their overall well-being. Before it is too late, we need to spread this valuable information to as many people as possible. Thank you, Dr. Siton, for writing our manual for optimal health!

— Dr. Nelson Valena, MD
Physiatrist
Physician Director of Rehabilitation
Nexus Neurorecovery Center

Gigi Siton, DPT, has truly given us a gift, a plethora of information on how to take care of ourselves. The extensive research behind all the topics that are discussed results in powerful new habits that can completely change our life! I highly recommend everyone to thoroughly read this book to give yourself a new lease on life and to achieve a happier and healthier future.

—Isabelle Valentine
CEO and Entrepreneur
Montessori Schools
Copenhagen, Denmark

Your Body Is a
SELF-HEALING
MACHINE

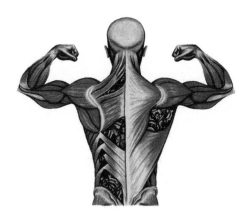

Your Body Is a
SELF-HEALING
M A C H I N E

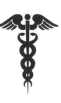

Understanding the Anatomy of Epigenetics
BOOK 2

Gigi Siton, DPT
Doctor of Physical Therapy

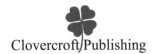

Clovercroft Publishing

Your Body Is a Self-Healing Machine: Understanding the Anatomy of Epigenetics, Book 2

©2021 Gigi Siton

Published by Clovercroft Publishing, Franklin, Tennessee

Edited by OnFire Books

Copy Edited by Lee Titus Elliott

Cover and Interior Design by Adept Content Solutions

Book Cover Graphics by Patrick Joven

Printed in the United States of America

ISBN: Hardcover 978-1-950892-85-3
      Trade Paperback 978-1-950892-83-9

*This book is lovingly dedicated
to the memory of my amazing parents:*

"Papa George" Attorney George Laurie Siton, Sr.

and

"Mama Liling" Eligia Flores Siton.

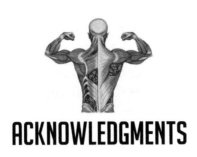

ACKNOWLEDGMENTS

Many people in my life have supported me, have believed in me, have given me hope, and have shared with me information that literally changed my life. The list would be extremely long, and I am limited for space, so thanks to everyone who continues to be part of my life. You know who you are. Thank you. Thank you. Thank you!

I would like to thank my beautiful daughters, Alexandra Siton Till and Victoria Siton Till, for being my inspiration in all that I do.

My thanks to the awesome Holistic Physical Therapy Team, Mylene Thormer BSN, Gary Picar PTA, Andrew Magahis, Tristan Bautista, Mini Puquiz, and Jennifer Osborne; without your unconditional support and commitment day in and day out, there would be no Holistic Physical Therapy Clinic. I thank you for helping people every day recapture their health, for believing and supporting my ideas and vision, and for making this company successful in making the world a healthier place to live!

I thank my dearest sister, Leah Siton Steigerwald, and her husband, Volker Steigerwald, PhD, who tirelessly edited this book while being quarantined in Germany. I thank Doods Siton and Ally Till for helping with book formatting. And, finally, I thank Lisa Capallia and Helen Conol for reviewing my book. I thank

Patrick J. Joven for drawing a masterpiece, the beautiful Self-Healing Body on the book cover.

To all my family and friends too many to mention, thank you for your support in my personal and professional life.

And, of course, I thank Mark Loughead, my biggest support, who got this book out of my head and into my hands.

Maraming Salamat Po!

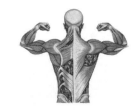

SERIES CONTENTS

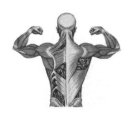

CONTENTS

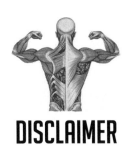

DISCLAIMER

This book is designed to provide helpful information on the subjects discussed. This book is not meant to be used, nor should it be used, to diagnose or to treat any psychological or medical condition. For diagnosis or treatment of any psychological or medical issue, consult your physician. The publisher and the author are not responsible for any specific health needs that may require medical supervision and are not liable for any damages or negative consequences from any treatment, action, application, or preparation to any person reading or following the information in this book. The author and the publisher refuse any and all warranties, liabilities, losses, costs, claims, demands, suits, and actions of any type or nature whatsoever, arising from or in any way related to this book. References are provided for informational purposes only and do not constitute an endorsement of any books, websites, or other sources. Readers should be aware that the websites listed in this book might change. Neither the publisher nor the author shall be liable for any physical, psychological, emotional, financial, or commercial damages, including, but not limited to, special, incidental, consequential, or other damages. The readers are responsible for their own choices, actions, and results.

Your Body Is a SELF-HEALING MACHINE

TRILOGY

Understanding the Anatomy of Epigenetics
BOOK 2

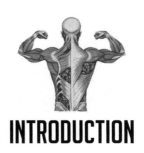

INTRODUCTION

Now that you have read Book One: *"Understanding Epigenetics—Why It Is Important to Know."* You know the basic concepts of epigenetics and why it is essential. Epigenetics shows us the way to heal our bodies and achieve a healthy existence. To move forward and restore our optimal health, we urgently need to update our medical systems. It is unbelievable that we are still stuck in the old conventional genetic code of victimhood for 100 years. Sadly, we have continued to take additional wrong paths at almost every opportunity, even today.

Fortunately, a new medical dawn is here. Epigenetics is the missing link that fills the blind spot of conventional medical science. Interestingly, there is nobody studying the combination of epigenetics with Western and Eastern medical healing concepts. Moving forward, the medical world needs to pool its knowledge into one comprehensive medical system.

Welcome to Book Two: *"Understanding the Anatomy of Epigenetics,"* the second book of the trilogy *YOUR BODY IS A SELF-HEALING MACHINE*. You are probably familiar with the basics of epigenetics by now after reading Book One: *"Understanding Epigenetics – Why It Is Important to Know."* You may be eager to get started in your healing practice. I do not blame you. I have found most of my patients are likely to succeed in self-healing when they understand the basics of epigenetic anatomy in the cells, the immune multisystems, the gut, and finally, the microbiota. Understanding your anatomy clears the path to knowing the root causes of poor health. I assume that you are eager to know where exactly epigenetics happens in your body. So, without further ado, Book Two will explain the basic nitty-gritty of your epigenetic anatomy.

Have you ever been told that everything you do affects every cell in your body? If you have, this book is for you. I will help you understand why you need to get familiar with the idea that your cell is the most critical citizen in your body. This book will cover why knowing your cell is essential—what it is made of, how it works, and its significant role in epigenetics. We will examine our cell's parts, the mitochondrial inputs and outputs within your cells, how your cell membranes cross communicate, and how your DNA and RNA are affected by epigenetics.

Also, we will cover your gut's digestion so that you will understand how your body's engine works. You will learn to appreciate that eighty percent of your immune system is in your stomach. We will discuss how to maintain a healthy gut and repair your gut if it is damaged. We will also discuss the basics of proper digestion, your digestive system's needs, and how essential stomach acids play a role in your health and immune system. Finally, we will discuss how to properly prepare nutrient-dense whole food, which our body requires to function to its optimal level.

Equally important, you will learn to appreciate your body's hardworking guest workers: your microbiota. When you know how to be an excellent host to your microbiome, you allow them to effectively aid in your body's health and heal any physical ailment. These are the massive bacterial and viral organisms that live in and on your body. You are composed of more microbes than human cells. This book will discuss how over-the-counter drugs, antacids, antibiotics, anti-histamines, and other non-steroidal anti-inflammatory drugs (NSAIDs) can adversely wreak havoc on your immune system by polluting your gut's microbiome.

In this book, I propose a new immune multisystem concept. It is essential to incorporate the autonomic nervous system, digestive system, lymphatic, and meridian systems to achieve efficient self-healing capabilities. I am convinced that this how it should be presented. In my medical training, the immune system was mentioned but not taught in a systematic way. It was never elevated as the most powerful system for optimal health. It is time to address our immune multisystem as our first line of defense against illness. More than ever, in this pandemic climate, we need to understand and master how to fortify or "bulletproof" your immune system against viral and bacterial infections.

I have incorporated applied epigenetics principles in my holistic PT practice and have witnessed patients' dramatic recoveries daily. As an example, let me share the results of a specific holistic physical therapy patient, a 64-year-old retired emergency room (ER) nurse named Miss Sheila K. She suffered from Reflex Sympathetic Dystrophy (RSD) Syndrome for 22 years, a devastating and painful injury sustained from a car accident. RSD is a chronic condition, most often following trauma to the extremities. It is characterized by severe burning pain, typically affecting one or more of the extremities (arms, legs, hands, or feet). The exact cause of RSD is not well understood but may involve abnormal inflammation or nerve dysfunction.

In my practice, it is always an exciting experience to work with chronic pain patients. I seem to be considered the last hope. The majority are jaded because they have tried conventional medicine for many years before they come to see me. Try to imagine my initial physical therapy evaluation session with Miss Sheila K: she hobbled with a straight cane into my examination room. I encountered a thin, frail woman hunched over to her left side, suffering in the agony of pain. I saw the angst in her eyes, a worn-out shell with the spirit of a warrior. The moment she sat down, her first line was: "You cannot fix me; I have RSD. I have been suffering constant, severe pain for 22 years, 24/7. Nothing has worked so far, but I am still alive." She said that her whole body felt like it was always on fire with burning pain with no relief. She presented with a chief complaint of constant severe burning pain, rated 9 out of 10 on her subjective pain scale, mostly on her body's left side than the right side. She was also taking medications for severe anxiety, insomnia, and depression. She had had to retire prematurely 20 years prior due to her dire unrelenting condition.

During her initial physical therapy evaluation, she struggled to get on the exam table. Her body's left side was severely weakened; her range of motion on both left upper and left lower extremities was less than 25 percent, with severe constant pain at rest. Her pain increased to 10 out of 10 with movement, even with a massive dose of multiple pain medications. She explained that she had been to many doctors all over the country and all the medical interventions you can name, but they had not helped her thus far. When we started our epigenetic approach to healing, Miss Sheila K was very resistant. I completely understood her skepticism. As an ER nurse, she embodied all the best conventional Western medicine had to offer. She had tried almost everything before—nearly everything except epigenetics with holistic foundational therapy. Despite her doubts and fears, she gave her full commitment to the Holistic Physical Therapy program.

We started with an extensive conversation about the importance of setting your brain in a healing mode – making a conscious choice to nurture a parasympathetic brain in addition to urgently addressing her digestive system. In just two weeks, with a properly prepared nutrient-dense diet and optimal hydration, she had a full range of her left upper and lower extremities, and her pain went down to 3 out of 10. Once she completed three weeks of extensive stimulation of her meridians and lymphatic systems, she could walk without her cane and participate in all her physical therapy exercise programs. I am super excited to report that she is now a renewed woman! She continues to practice the epigenetics approach to health and healing. She takes no medications and still uses food as medicine. She is pain-free in all her joints, walks three miles daily, dances, volunteers, and works around her neighborhood to help other people. She even expressed that she was so surprised by her brain function.

She can tell that her long-term memory and short-term recall function again, and her anxiety is almost gone. She is sleeping better and better every day. She continues to make significant improvements and is so much happier now. Every time she comes to the clinic, she sashays with cool outfits and smiles ear-to-ear! Amazingly after 23 years, she is thinking of restarting her medical career. My Holistic PT team and I have seen epigenetics work repeatedly for thousands of patients in our holistic physical therapy clinic. The best part is that epigenetics is useful for permanent healing. This story and thousands of others make my medical profession so worthwhile.

Rewarding as Miss Sheila K's story sounds, allow me to begin sharing with you the second book of the trilogy ***"Your Body Is A Self-Healing Machine"*: Understanding The Anatomy of Epigenetics.**

It is time to start your story, so let us begin.

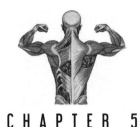

CHAPTER 5
WHERE IS THE EPICENTER OF EPIGENETICS?

"Everyone has a physician inside him or her;
we just have to help it in its work."
—Hippocrates

THE CELL

ANIMAL CELL ANATOMY

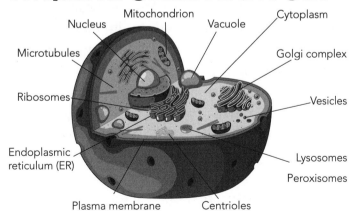

FIGURE 2.1. Cell Anatomy

1

Life and health begin and end at the cell level of our body. Our cells are our building blocks. They are our foundation. According to Dr. Bill Cole, MD, Key Cellular Nutrition (KCN), all human body functions come from our cells. That means that any type of dysfunction, that is, symptoms that a person might have or even any full-blown disease, is always traceable back to something gone wrong at the body's cellular level.

The epicenter of epigenetics is located in your cell. Your cell is the fundamental core unit in your body where all epigenetic interactions happen. You can think of your cell as an individual citizen that lives in your body's community. According to Dr. Mark Atkinson, MD, PhD, Professor of Medicine, University of Florida, *"The human body is a tight community of 100 trillion cells. It is essential to keep every cell healthy."*[1]

Your cell is the basic structure of the human body. Your body's cells are classified according to individual cell functions. Once individual cells share a joint task, they bond together. These grouped cells become a tissue; arranged tissues function together, comprising organs. Grouped organs share joint function and develop into a system. A grouping of this system of organs makes up the body.

There are many different types, sizes, and shapes of cells in the body. Every tissue, every organ, every gland, every body part is made of cells, whether it is skin cells or bone cells or heart cells or thyroid cells or blood cells or even the cells of our immune system like our while blood cells. With that in mind, knowing that cells are our foundation, we need to make sure that each cell is healthy. If our cells are not functioning in any part of our body, we cannot be healthy. In this section, we will know our cell parts and what it needs.

Your cell anatomy has three main parts: the cell membrane, the nucleus, and, between the two, the cytoplasm.

Concepts about a cell structure's importance have changed considerably over the years. In the past, it was overemphasized that the nucleus is the most essential part of the cell. However, your cell membrane and mitochondria should be given more significance than they have been given historically. Your nucleus may house your DNA, but your cell can live without the nucleus. Yet, the cell *will* immediately expire if you remove the cell membrane. Besides, if your mitochondria malfunction, it will affect your gene expression. As a result, you are more likely to get sick quickly and may not recover well due to mitochondria or membrane changes, rather than nucleus changes. It is crucial for you to have practical information about every single-cell unit, specifically how to grow, maintain, fortify, and, finally, repair your cell when broken. Your cell's epigenetics information (comprised of your cell's environment, your cell's foundational nutrition, and your cell's self-healing mechanisms) is the main factor in your cell's gene expression.

HOMEOSTASIS

What is homeostasis? It comes from two Greek words: "homeo," meaning "similar," and "stasis," meaning "stable." Homeostasis means a stable, balanced state of equilibrium within a cell or elsewhere within the body. This is your body's optimal goal 24/7: maintaining a stable and balanced internal environment. This requires constant adjustments for your body, as conditions change inside and outside every cell within your body. The primary gatekeepers for homeostasis are the two walls or layers of your cell membrane. Homeostasis entails balancing cells, maintaining an equilibrium of ions and molecules swimming within the cells and outside the cells.

THE NUCLEUS

The nucleus has been considered the control center of the cell because it houses our genes. Its wall is called a "nuclear membrane"; the nucleus's fluids are called the "nucleoplasm." Within the core of the nucleus is the nucleolus. It is in the nucleolus where you can find the chromosome's genetic material of your cell, which is made up of deoxyribonucleic acid (DNA) and ribonucleic acid (RNA).

Your cell's core is the keeper of your DNA blueprint for all cell functions. It is also here that the histone-wrapping response takes place. A *histone* is a protein that provides structural support to a chromosome. For very long DNA molecules to fit into the cell nucleus, they wrap around complexes of histone proteins, giving the chromosome a more compact shape. Variation in the quality of the histones wrapping is associated with the regulation of gene expression. Its protein integrity is affected by epigenetics' environmental composition in the nucleoplasm.

According to Dr. William A. Gahl, MD, PhD, geneticist, Clinical Director of the National Human Genome Research Institute at the NIH, *"Histones are proteins that are critical in the packing of DNA into the cell and chromatin and chromosomes. They're also very important for the regulation of genes. We used to think that histones acted essentially as DNA suitcases to sort of hold the DNA, but it was obvious that histones are regulated and have a lot to do with when genes are turned on and turned off. You can think about them as a regulated suitcase that determines when the suitcase is opened, and a gene gets out. So, they turn out to have very*

CELL MEMBRANE

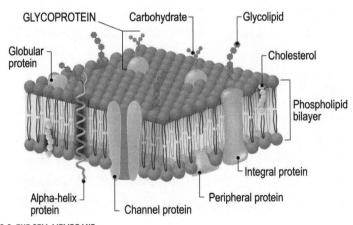

FIGURE 2.2. THE CELL MEMBRANE

important functions, not only structurally, but also in the regulation of gene function in the expression."[2]

THE CELL MEMBRANE

The cell membrane, or cell wall, is also known as the plasma membrane. Your cell membrane is your biological border, or wall, that separates the interior of all the cell's organs from the outside environment.

It is interesting to examine the word "membrane." Initially, I thought it was an old English spelling. However, after reading this from Bruce Lipton, PhD, it made sense that the "brane" in "membrane" could be considered as the "brain" of the cells. "*Cellular life is sustained by tightly regulating the functions of the cell's physiologic systems. The expression of predictable behavioral repertoires implies the existence of a cellular nervous system.*"[3] This system reacts to environmental stimuli by eliciting appropriate behavioral responses. The organelle that coordinates the adjustments and reactions of a cell to its internal and external environments would represent the cytoplasmic equivalent of the brain. Therefore, the cell membrane is the brain or the primary driver of all cell functions. It also acts as the eyes, ears, and skin of your cells. "*Without the cell membranes, life as we know it would not be possible,*" according to Steven R. Goodman, PhD, vice chancellor for the University of Tennessee Health Science (UTHSC) Research, Medical Cell Biology.[4]

Your cell membrane has the powerful function of controlling what can come in and out of the cell to maintain both liquids and solids' homeostasis. One of the great wonders of the cell membrane is its ability to regulate the concentration of substances inside the cell. These substances include ions, such as calcium ($Ca++$), sodium ($Na+$), potassium ($K+$), and chloride ($Cl-$); nutrients, including sugars, fatty acids, amino acids, and waste products, particularly carbon dioxide (CO^2), which must leave the cell.[5]

The cell membrane illustration in Figure 2.2 is a simplified version of the more extensive cell membrane, with its corresponding intricate and extensive bio-cellular structures. The cell membrane's lipid bilayer structure provides the first level of control. It has two layers of fats, called phospholipids. "Phospho" comes from the molecule phosphate, while "lipids" are the molecular fats. Phospholipids are simply phosphate + fats. It should be clarified that molecular fats or lipids in your cell membrane are the broken elements of essential fatty acids from the good healthy fats you eat. The most abundant primary raw materials in the outer layer of the cell membrane are phospholipids. These two layers serve as a flexible and robust skin casing of the cell membrane that holds all the other cell structures in place.

The cell membrane's shape, stability, and flexibility are dependent on the health of the phospholipids. The cell membrane lipid bilayers consist of saturated fatty acids and unsaturated fatty acids. This combination comprises, in part, the fluidity of the cell membrane, which is continuously in motion.

Given that your cells' primary fortification is made mainly of water and fats, it is critical to eat good-quality healthy fats daily for your cell membrane's health.[6] For the past sixty years, the miseducation on fat-free diets and fat phobias have wreaked havoc on our basic cell-membrane structure. A diet without good fats is like a house with weak walls. We cannot expect paper-thin walls to stand against wind and water; it is the same in a diet without healthy fats. Fats fortify the cell membrane as brick fortifies a house.[7] Find more on fats in Book Three.

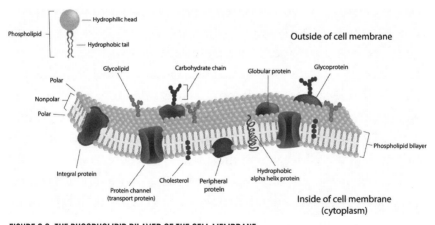

FIGURE 2.3. THE PHOSPHOLIPID BILAYER OF THE CELL MEMBRANE

The phospholipid layers are fat cell walls that have two opposites but complementary functions between the two layers. This has to do with their behavioral response to water. The phospholipid bilayer that forms the cell surface membrane consists of a hydrophobic inner core region sandwiched between two hydrophilicity areas. The inner core or inside surface blocks water, while the outside surface loves water. Its primary function is to hold enough water inside to maintain balance or homeostasis.

Let us discuss in more depth the importance of the cell-wall structure and its water response. The inside of the phospholipid layer is hydrophobic. "Hydro" from Greek means water, while "phobic," from the word phobia, means strong dislike. They are uncharged, or nonpolar, and are hydrophobic—or water-fearing. A hydrophobic molecule (or region of a molecule) repels and is repelled by water. That means it stops more water from coming in or leaving once enough water inside the cell is detected. This inner core prevents unnecessary leaking of the fluids, mainly water and minerals, once inside the cell membrane wall.

The outer fat layer of the cell membrane is hydrophilic. Again, "hydro" refers to water, while "-philic" means a fondness for a specific thing. The phosphate group is negatively charged, making the head polar and hydrophilic—or water-loving. A hydrophilic molecule is one that is attracted to water. The phosphate heads (as seen as the red round balls in the illustration Figure 2.3) are attracted to the water molecules of both the extracellular (outside the cell) and intracellular (inside the cell) environments. It is selective as to how much water goes in and out of the cell membrane by osmosis or the gradient difference is maintained.

These different functions make the cell membrane very efficient, allowing it to discriminate what will enter and what will exit. This function is known as selective permeability. One of the primary contents of the cell membrane is water. Water serves as the filler and the primary medium where most ions and molecules reside. The cell communication highway runs between the phospholipid layers. It is like the main freeway of nutrient exchange and communication between cells and between systems.

The cell membrane also serves as a shock absorber between the cells. When it is fully filled with water, the membrane expands and thickens the cell wall. It becomes efficient in absorbing any external shock to protect the inside and outside surrounding structures from damage.

Approximately 80 percent of the cell membrane is water. This emphasizes the importance of proper hydration in our bodily functions. According to Dr. Fereydoon Batmanghelidj, MD, water is the preferred hydration for your body. It also needs the eighty-nine minerals which can be found in ancient sea salt. The mineral electrolytes energize the water with electrical charges. Effectively, it helps open the cell membrane to let the water molecules enter the cells.

If this feels like a lot of information, you should know that there is almost nothing more valuable than studying the way your body functions. There are so many myths and such a massive body of misinformation. In these pages, I have worked hard to provide you with the most important details about your health. Too many people are misinformed, even on seemingly simple concepts such as hydration; not enough people drink enough water to replenish and restore their cells properly!

Fluids other than water are a burden to your kidney. Your kidney must work harder to separate water from every drink that is not water, eventually leading to dehydration because of the extra work the kidney is doing.[8] Unintended chronic dehydration is the fundamental enemy of the cell membrane. We will discuss the importance of water more in Chapter 11 of Book Three.

The lipid bilayer forms the basis of the cell membrane, but the membrane also contains various proteins. The integral and peripheral proteins in the cell membrane are the entrance points or gates for all molecules on their way inside the cell's cytoplasm or the cell's inner ocean. You need to have the right key in the proper enzymes or micronutrients to open these entry points. The cell membrane is very selective as to which ions and molecules are allowed entry. Once opened, the membrane also controls the amount of movement of substances in and out of cells. It is the chief gatekeeper of the traffic flow of particles to maintain cell homeostasis. A healthy cell membrane lets nutrients in and toxins out with the proper enzymes and micronutrients for optimal health. In contrast, a blocked or breached gate of the cell membrane is a disease symptom, irrespective of the cell function.

"Peripheral" or *outlying* proteins act as the windows and the doors along the walls of your cell membrane. Your cell membrane's doors and windows require keys in the form of the right enzymes to unlock and open their respective peripheral membrane proteins. The specific keys or protein enzymes will open and let the necessary ions and molecules in or out, depending on what the body needs at a given moment. Oligosaccharides can have many functions, including cell recognition and cell binding. Glycolipids have an essential role in the cell membrane's strength and aid in cell identification, which is useful for immune response. Also, it allows cells to connect to form tissues. Glycoproteins are simply proteins with molecular sugar in the form of glucose attached to them. They are usually on the outside of the cell membrane, with the sugar facing out. Glycoproteins participate in almost all cell processes. They have an essential role in our immune system, protecting our body, exchanging information between cells and our reproductive system. Glycoproteins in your red blood cells identify your blood type. They help the body recognize that your blood is a part of you, and they tell it not to attack it. Glycoproteins also help trigger the thickening process to clot your blood when you get cut.

Your cell membrane has highly efficient physical properties: biomechanical, biochemical, and bioelectrical. First, the *biomechanical property* refers to the cell wall's physical behavior when forces are applied to it. Examples of these mechanical or physical properties are as follows: (1) elasticity: how flexible the cell wall is; (2) tensile strength: what the breaking strength of the cell wall is after an applied force or just after normal wear and tear; (3) cell elongation: how much permanent increase there is in the surface of the cell wall; and (4) fatigue limit, also known as "endurance limit" or "fatigue strength": that is, how much stress the cell wall sustains before it fails. These bio-structural properties of the cell wall affect living cells' behavior and their relation to cell function.

Second, the *cell wall's biochemical components* come basically from molecules of fats, water, sugars, and proteins. They are located along the fatty walls of the cells. They are composed mostly of fats and proteins. These wall sensors serve as message couriers, using the right enzymes and receptors to relay the necessary information between cells throughout the body.

Third and finally, the *bioelectrical properties* come with biochemical reactions. According to neurobiologist Daniel Kirsch, PhD, the inventor of Alpha-Stim, *"Electrical activity precedes chemical activity and controls it."* All the biochemical messages involved bioelectrical signals first.[9] Your cell membrane has an intrinsic electromagnetic field that allows optimizing bioelectrical cell function. Your body needs to maintain an optimal bioelectrical charge in your cell membrane to facilitate all the physiological functions which follow. Without electricity in your cell membrane, nothing happens. It is critical to be aware of this and be proactive about protecting your cell membrane's bioelectrical health. This means avoiding exposure to toxic metals, as well as to toxic EMFs, which can have a dire impact on your cell membrane, as well as on your mitochondria—more on bioelectrical properties in Chapter 6 "Cell Voltage."

THE CYTOPLASM

The word "cytoplasm" originates from a combination of two words: "cyto," from the ancient Greek word "kutos," which means "vessel," and "plasm," from the ancient Greek word "plassein," which means "to shape." The cytoplasm is the gel-like liquid or the ocean inside the cell, where most cell diffusion or molecular cell movement happens. Biological cell diffusion is a process by which molecules can move into or out of the cell, going from a higher concentration to a lower concentration. It is how the chemical reaction happens in the cell. This is where new cell functions such as expansion, growth, and replication are carried out.

THE MITOCHONDRIA

Many exciting epigenetic reactions happen inside your mitochondria. Your mitochondria are shaped like miniature submarine capsules swimming in the cytoplasm inside the cell. Usually, according to that particular cell's function, there are hundreds to thousands of mitochondria per cell. Your mitochondria are like the microcellular version of the triple-A battery with bioelectrical output. Your mighty mitochondria are the potent batteries that power your cells. Mitochondria are the primary producers of cell energy, which is why they are also called "the powerhouse of the cell."

To grasp the sheer scale of the impact of mitochondria on our overall health, consider this: each of us has quadrillions (that is, thousands of trillions) of these energy factories in our bodies. On average, every cell has 1,500 mitochondria. Nerve cells have 4,500-to-6,000 mitochondria, and some cells have many more.[10] Dr. Gottfried Schatz, PhD, called the mitochondria a *"Magic Garden: one billion of your mitochondria would fit in a grain of sand, yet, gram for gram, your mitochondria convert between 10,000 and 50,000 times more energy per second than the sun."*[11] Just as your car needs the power to move the engine, so does your body need power from your mitochondria to crank up all the individual cells in your body. If your mitochondria have no power, at first, you will be fatigued. If your mitochondria are ignored or poisoned by a lousy diet, you will then become sick, and you may develop what is called "mitochondrial dysfunction."

Mitochondria are powered by oxygen. The mitochondria are the cell organs for respiration. It is the lungs of your cell. Your cells use mitochondria to process oxygen. Your mitochondria also generate a massive number of harmful waste products, called free radicals. This is the site where the most significant amount of reactive oxygen species in our bodies exists. The paradox is that while you cannot exist without oxygen, oxygen is also inherently dangerous to your existence because each oxygen atom has an unpaired electron in its outer valence shell. Without sufficient antioxidants to pair with them, these electrons produce oxygen toxicity. Examples of such toxicity include the superoxide anion radical, hydrogen peroxide, and the extremely reactive hydroxyl radical.[12]

Your mitochondria are the tiny factories in each of our cells that turn the food we eat and the oxygen we breathe into energy. Hans Krebs discovered how cells produce energy in the mitochondrial biochemical process called the "Krebs cycle." The cycle needs oxygen, water, vitamin C, ketones, glucose, zinc, and other minerals.

Your mighty mitochondria use both biochemical and bioelectrical processes to perform their biological job. They produce the cell's main power for cell-energy production, cell respiration, adenosine triphosphate (ATP)-cell-energy production; they also maintain glutathione levels, protect DNA, signal cell reproduction, activate cell apoptosis, and maintain cell-electrochemical integrity.

Each mitochondrion is filled with approximately 17,000 biochemical assembly lines. All of your mitochondria are designed to produce an ATP molecule, our body's major, most elemental fuel.[13] It is the molecule that our cells use as energy. The mitochondria store your body's supply of ATP, like rechargeable batteries.

Your mitochondria also hold many protein enzymes essential for cell metabolism. Also, they maintain the cell's electrochemical integrity. They are responsible for supplying your cell membrane with its electrical voltage level so that the cell is always ready to perform consistent biochemical and bioelectrical reactions to maintain overall health.

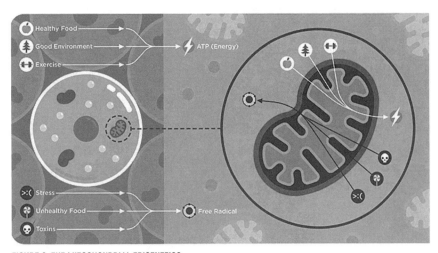

FIGURE 9. THE MITOCHONDRIAL EPIGENETICS

How do epigenetic factors affect your mitochondria? It is in your mitochondria where the "rubber meets the road" 'in epigenetics. Your mitochondria hold and protect your genetic protein, the mitochondrial DNA genes. In the mitochondria, the methyl groups actively tag your genes for expression, that is, flagging them to either be turned on or to be silenced. In your mitochondria, epigenetic activities are manipulating your gene expression and reading your DNA blueprint. Whenever your cell membrane lets in a molecule, your mitochondria use it to produce power for the cell, as well as to "reset" or to "update" your gene "software." Suppose you provide your mitochondria with the best raw molecules from the environment outside, such as healthy food and a healthy, healing mind-set. In that case, your genetic software will be updated accordingly. Your genetic potential blueprint is expressed as a response to the biochemical signals from the epigenetic environment surrounding it. An example of such an environment would include healthy fats, an active lifestyle, and positive coping mechanisms. Epigenetics reprograms DNA gene expression in your mitochondria. Your epigenetics choices stimulate mitochondrial responses, which affect your health either positively or negatively.

Your mitochondria are also responsible for signaling the body to reproduce new cells when they are signaled to do so by the outside environment. Additionally, they trigger weak or sick cells to die (a process called "apoptosis"), so these cells do not clog up the body.

What can damage your mitochondria? Mitochondrial dysfunction can be caused by stress, infections, toxins, nutrient deficiencies, specific treatments such as chemotherapy, irradiation, pesticides, chemicals, poor lifestyle, EMF overexposure, unhealthy diet (too much sugar or too much protein), microbes (viruses or bacteria), overexposure to the sun, poor sleeping habits, and dehydration. All these factors can weaken your mitochondria. Your body's physiology, while under stress, can use up much of your cells ATP energy fuel and can prevent cell reproduction and repair. It will eventually cause mitochondrial genome breakdown, dysfunction, and disease.

According to mitochondrial health advocate Dr. Terry Wahls, MD, healthy fats are the preferred fuel for the mitochondria; Dr. Wahls reversed her multiple sclerosis diagnosis with a ketogenic diet.[14] She has actively supported a diet of healthy fats. Healthy fats protect mitochondria by providing anti-inflammatory support. While the mitochondria can use *either* fatty acids or carbohydrates to produce energy, healthy fats allow mitochondria to work more efficiently and create fewer free-radical byproducts. Healthy fats can come from oily fish in your diet, avocados, coconut oil, olive oil, or flaxseed oil—more on fats in Book Three

Beware of sugar! It will slow down the cell-energy production in your mitochondria.[15] The empty calories of sugars, flours, and other processed foods force mitochondria to burn through a great deal of junk—generating free radicals and inflammation as they go—before useful nutrients can be extracted.[16]

It is vital to maintain fully charged mitochondria for optimal health. Electrochemical energy comes from the food you eat and the correct epigenetic information from your healthy choices. Therefore, the mitochondria require a diet rich in antioxidants. This includes colorful vegetables, fruit, herbs and spices, and other healthy foods that supply essential nutrients. Your mitochondria also need a healthy supply of properly prepared nutrient-dense whole foods from organic, pasture-raised meat, wild-caught fish, nuts, seeds, beans (like lentils), and eggs and pasture-raised chickens for complete amino acids support—more on healthy food in Book 3.

Your mitochondria also need two specific antioxidants: alpha-lipoic acid and coenzyme Q10. Alpha-lipoic acid is found in spinach, broccoli, yams, potatoes, yeast, tomatoes, Brussels sprouts, carrots, beets, and rice bran. Red meat—particularly organ meat—is also a source of alpha-lipoic acid. These antioxidants support the efficient reproduction of your mitochondria and the renewal of mitochondrial cells. The more mitochondria, the more cell power! They need micronutrients for energy production, mostly from vitamin C. Additional vitamins are also required, such as vitamin E, vitamin B, magnesium, iron, and selenium.

Since your mitochondria are the leading suppliers of the cell's electrical charges, they are susceptible to damage from an electromagnetic field. A 2019 scientific study investigated smartphones' daily use of nonionizing low-frequency electromagnetic waves (NLFEW) for fifteen days and their adverse health effects on a chick embryo.[17] The study concluded that daily exposure to NLFEW caused early damage to mitochondria in the liver and a chick embryo's heart tissues.[17] Consistent external electrical disruption from any Wi-Fi source will more than likely change the polarity charge of your mitochondria. Eventually, a low-voltage mitochondrion will cause cells to become sick. Mitochondria are sensitive to toxins, which can exist in medications and chemicals which may block mitochondrial function.[18]

Consistent healthy-gut detoxification is vital for mitochondrial health; it is like a regular house cleaning for the mitochondria. We will discuss more on detoxification in Book Three.

 Epigenetics changes happen in your nucleus and in your mitochondria. Your cell membrane controls what comes in and out of your cells.

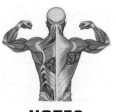

NOTES

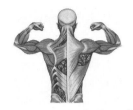

CHAPTER 6
YOUR BODY'S SELF-HEALING SYSTEMS

"If someone wishes for good health, one must first ask oneself if he is ready to do away with the reasons for his illness. Only then is it possible to help him."
—Hippocrates

Are you ready to take charge of your health? If you are ready to practice the new habits discussed in the following chapter, I guarantee that you will feel better and stronger and see a big difference in your look and feel. This chapter will introduce a novel concept that is outside the box of mainstream Western medicine. When I was a physical therapy student and psychology student many moons ago, I was taught a reductionist model in the study of the human body. Each system was very compartmentalized and isolated from one another. The connection of each system's physiology was taught but downplayed. In other words, the reductionist model was not an integrative approach. Sadly, the current practice of conventional Western medicine has divided each system according to its respective specialist. Each medical specialty has a boundary to separate it from the next specialty. Since the 1930s, conventional Western medicine has chosen a minimal approach to biochemical and surgical interventions.

These conventional teachings are the opposite of the comprehensive approach of ancient medical systems that exist in Asia. The Ayurveda, TCM, the Philippine manual-massage approach called "Hilot," and herbal and nutritional medicine practiced in other parts of the world are a few examples of this comprehensive approach. In these ancient medical systems, the human body's study is more integrated as one whole system, interconnected with its environment's biorhythm. For thousands of years, these ancient medical systems were practicing the principles of "applied epigenetics," even before the term was invented.

THE IMMUNE MULTISYSTEM

This section will expand on this concept of the profound inter-connectedness of our body's systems. I propose that the immune system is actually multisystem within the body. It depends on multiple factors which, in a healthy body, work together efficiently. Each part has a significant function in the processes of self-healing and recovery.

Your immune multisystem works similarly to the way a car engine does. A car engine has several internal parts that work together to produce the power that moves the vehicle. For the engine to operate correctly, all its parts need to be in good condition. One fault can be disastrous.

You can look at your health through a new lens that will enable you to understand this immune multisystem better and find a way forward to improve your health. Your biological self-healing engine comprises five major systems that work together to make up an efficient immune multisystem. In this chapter, I suggest a change to the immune system's components as they have been understood in Western medicine. Going forward, we may understand the components in terms of the Meridians in Traditional Chinese medicine (TCM), the Autonomic Nervous System (ANS), the Endocannabinoid System (ECS), the Lymphatic System, and the Digestive System.

This perspective repudiates how many conventional mainstream medicines view your immune system. First, according to this approach, the primary driver of your immune multisystem is located in the ANS within your brain and spinal cord. Knowing the brain's setting for healing, the parasympathetic system, is very critical. Second, your immune system requires optimal electrical supply within your body to power it. This is why it is vital to know your body's electrical wiring. Your body's electrical system is laid out according to the TCM meridians network. Third, your endocannabinoid system is "the new kid in the block" as far as medical science is discovering its presence in your brain and the rest of your body. ECS helps us maintain homeostasis by monitoring what is going on in our bodies. Fourth, your lymphatic system's role in your immune system is to transport fat-soluble vitamins throughout the body. It is also your body's plumbing for protective cells and defensive cell armies against invaders like bacteria and viruses. Finally, your digestive system is where the raw materials, like food, are processed to supply the necessary parts and fuel your main body engine and your immune system.

Most people have no idea precisely what composes our immune system or how it works. Through traditional Western courses of study, I learned the reductionist way of looking at the different body systems: the muscular system, the skeletal system, the circulatory system, the respiratory system, the nervous system, the cardiac system, and the lymphatic system (which, by the way, was not taught in enough detail). There was no emphasis on the mechanism or the cooperation of the immune multisystem.

In this chapter, I will highlight the intricate beauty of the immune multisystem. It helps to understand why we are a self-healing organism when we recognize our body's divine design.

THE AUTONOMIC NERVOUS SYSTEM

It is essential to understand the autonomic nervous system (ANS) because it controls the body's general state at any given time. Imagine your brain setting as a radio set. Just as you have a choice as to which radio station to listen to (between the FM and the AM broadcasting systems), you have a choice as to which of your brain's ANS systems to set for your physiology, according to your state of mind. Your ANS has two systems: (1) the sympathetic nervous system, also known as the *"fight-or-flight"* system, and (2) the parasympathetic nervous system, or the *"rest-and-repair"* system.

Your ANS is a control system that mostly acts unconsciously and regulates bodily functions, such as heart rate, digestion, respiratory rate, pupillary response, urination, and sexual arousal. It is primarily designed for your protection and survival. The body

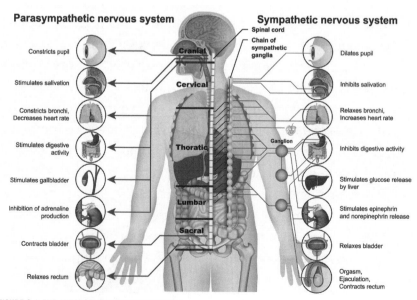

FIGURE 2.4. THE AUTONOMIC NERVOUS SYSTEM

functions may be automatic in your ANS, but the state of your mind greatly affects the ANS setting on which your body will run. According to Bruce H. Lipton, PhD, *"Our beliefs control our bodies, our minds, and thus our lives."*[19] Put differently, and your beliefs run your biology. Knowing how your organs function within each system is extremely important in understanding your general health. Your subjective perceptions and responses to environmental signals control the ANS setting on which your body will function. This knowledge can empower you to work with your body and your mind to achieve optimal health.

The Sympathetic Nervous System

The sympathetic nervous system, or the *"flight-or-fight"* system, is our automatic stress-response mechanism for protection and survival. Anthropologically, this has been our innate warning system for the human species to survive in the wild. When humans were hunters and gatherers, the sympathetic nervous system helped us to sense danger before it happened. (Perhaps, our "sixth sense" or "gut feeling" originated from the sympathetic nervous system.) When, for example, we encountered a saber-toothed tiger, the shock and the stress of the encounter would activate our sympathetic nervous system. The sympathetic nervous system enables us to decide whether to defend ourselves from imminent danger or run from it.

Biologically, once a threat or stress is detected, whether real or imagined, it suspends all the body's healing and growth processes. Your body activates the stress response and produces the hormone cortisol, known as the *stress hormone*, to set your body into survival mode. In this state, your stomach contracts, and no effective digestion can happen because survival is the priority. It is not the time for eating and relaxing. Digestion becomes complicated and inefficient because no saliva or gastric acids are produced. Reproduction is suspended; having babies while in this stress mode is impossible. The heart will beat faster, while blood pressure rises to pump necessary blood to the legs and extremities so that you can run more quickly from danger. Your pancreas will crank up more insulin in the blood just in case your muscles need it in preparation for the *fight-or-flight* response. Your brain will be vigilantly awake, scanning for danger, so that restorative sleep is impossible. No sleep means your body will not repair, and therefore cannot efficiently defend your health from invading microbes, whether bacterial or viral, because it is busy merely trying to survive.

Until the perceived or real danger or stress is gone, your body will be in survival mode. However, the body can only tolerate short bursts of the sympathetic mode. Once it receives a cue from your brain that the danger is gone, the stress reaction will stop. When you calm your mind with healthy coping mechanisms, such as the practices of prayer and meditation, your sympathetic autonomic nervous system will switch to the parasympathetic mode or the "healing mode." The cue could signify a real absence of physical danger, or it could be the absence of your subjective perception of stress. Such threats can also arouse you into a defensive action if you encounter something that alarms or enrages you. In modern-day situations, that alarming or enraging feeling can stem from perceived mental or emotional stresses, such as depression, financial anxiety, rejection, a traffic jam, or even a bad social media tweet, rather than from a real danger of a saber-toothed tiger.

Consider this: if you quickly scan your sympathetic physiology (left side of Figure 2.4), it describes many medical conditions. A prolonged sympathetic nervous response wll likely lead to *sympathetic overload syndrome.* Most chronic degenerative diseases are caused by sympathetic overload syndrome. Under stress, the sympathetic nervous system is always switched on and unable to turn itself off. It gives rise to a host of physical disorders such as chronic muscle pain, irritable bowel syndrome (IBS), cardiac disease, and even cancer. Stress hormones associated with this problem also degrade the function of pleasure centers contained within the brain.

Anxiety disorders are the psychological manifestations of the chronically aroused sympathetic nervous system. These can be dangerous. An extreme example of this is the *general adaptation syndrome*. It is an enlargement of the adrenal gland, atrophy of the thymus, spleen, and other lymphoid tissue, including gastric ulcerations. This is a lethal clinical problem that emerges from mental and physical exhaustion caused by the ravages of a relentless *fight-or-flight* response. This sounds like a close cousin of chronic fatigue syndrome.

General adaptation syndrome was discovered by Hans Selye, a student at Johns Hopkins University and McGill University, and a researcher at Université de Montréal. Selye described three adaptation stages, including an initial brief alarm reaction, followed by a prolonged resistance period, ending in a terminal stage of exhaustion and death. He experimented with animals by putting them under different physical and mental adverse conditions and noted that, under these severe conditions, the body consistently adapted to heal and recover.[20]

An individuals' healthy survival will likely depend on merely developing suitable coping mechanisms. Your body's immune system is very literal in responding to stress, whether perceived or actual. Therefore, it is crucial to consider how you interpret your daily situation; is a given threat real or perceived? Your conscious interpretation of and response to your daily life determines whether or not your body will activate the stress response. Without your conscious input, your body will have the same physiological response to a stress stimulus regardless of its gravity. It does not matter whether you are stuck in traffic, missing a deadline, or going through a divorce.

We need to master how to calm ourselves down in both a small and large crisis. The first line of defense against sympathetic overload is breathing. We tend to hold our breath when under stress, which leads to a decrease of oxygen flowing into our brain. Mild hypoxia will trigger your mind into *fight-or-flight* mode. It is essential to reset your stress stimulus standard to maintain your body in a parasympathetic mode.

In contrast, we may also define our standards of joy. We must consciously choose to celebrate and exaggerate joyful feelings on small events daily. Choosing to be a positive thinker is like consciously setting your brain to parasympathetic mode, the *"rest and relax"* mode. This will trigger a proportionate physiological response; it is not just a mental exercise. Gratitude is the best antidote to anxiety and depression.

I suggested defining a stressful situation in a more specific and literal way in my applied epigenetics class. Redefining your interpretation of stress in your life protects your brain from being in constant survival mode. I suggest using the word *stress* only in situations wherein your oxygen supply is about to be cut off. Anything below that is just a challenge, whether you are stuck in traffic, missing a deadline, or going through a divorce. None of these things will cut off your oxygen supply. You do not have to be in a sustained sympathetic drive. You can overcome it; just breathe!

The Parasympathetic Nervous System

The second system of the ANS is the Parasympathetic Nervous System (PNS), also called the *rest-and-digest* system or the *repair-and-heal* system. It is the ideal brain setting for active growth and healing to occur. It is possible in many circumstances to *choose* to be in a more relaxed or nonthreatened state. To be in a parasympathetic state is mostly internal, an active conscious decision not dependent on external cues. The expression, "Be the eye of the hurricane instead of the wall, where the most destruction occurs," applies here. The storm's eye is the calmest; more importantly, it is the hurricane path driver.

Endorphins or *"anti-cortisol hormones"* and healthy gastric enzymes are produced only during the parasympathetic state. A relaxed stomach is ready for effective digestion. Deep sleep will be possible, and anxiety and other psychological disorders can heal within the brain. The heart will relax, and blood pressure will normalize. The reproduction will become possible, and peripheral muscles and bones will be more efficient. Your immune system will be at its optimal level in a parasympathetic state.

Prayer or meditation, specifically contemplative and repetitive prayers, keep one in the parasympathetic mode. The psychophysiology of repetitive prayer is found in almost all ancient religions. A growing body of evidence-based research at Harvard Medical School and the Mind/Body Medical Institute at Deaconess Hospital suggests that repetitive prayer techniques, such as the Jesus Prayer, may offset the psychological and physiological wear and tear of our stressful lives.[21] Prayer first thing in the morning and before bedtime keeps your daily rhythm in a relaxed mode. Prayer before meals cues your brain and your gut to reset into parasympathetic mode. Prayer before meals is ideal for optimal digestion.

It is also significant to note that, during meals, a sitting position in a relaxed setting promotes better digestion in a parasympathetic mode without distractions, such as watching TV or working on the computer. It is the custom in most Asian countries to sit on the floor while eating, a practice that gets you closer to the earth and sets the parasympathetic mode more efficiently.

Oxytocin is known as the hormone that promotes feelings of love, bonding, and well-being. A 2018 study on oxytocin methylation was associated only with the autonomic nervous system's parasympathetic branch and was found present only at times of rest.[22] This study highlighted the importance of the oxytocin system's epigenetic regulation in anxiety-related and fear-related processes. The oxytocin methylation activates the "antistress hormone" in people.

THE MERIDIAN SYSTEM—YOUR BODY'S ELECTRICAL CIRCUIT

Medical science generally accepts the dynamic nature of life. This understanding is evident in the hospital. There is the use of electrocardiographs (ECGs) and electromyography (EMGs). They show us the intrinsic bioelectrical nature of the human body. Put simply, without the bioelectrical nature of the human body, there are no signs of life. With it, there are signs of life! All chemical reactions in the body are mediated first by its electrical signals. Electrical activity always precedes chemical action.

Most ancient healing practices in the world are aware of the power of our body's bioelectrical functions. Meridian healing is one of the oldest healing processes in ancient medical science. The meridians are a set of energy pathways in the body, where vital bioelectrical energy flows. According to TCM, the body's meridians are a network of *energy channels* or *qi* (life force; literally, vital breath). They are also called *prana* in the Ayurveda traditions.

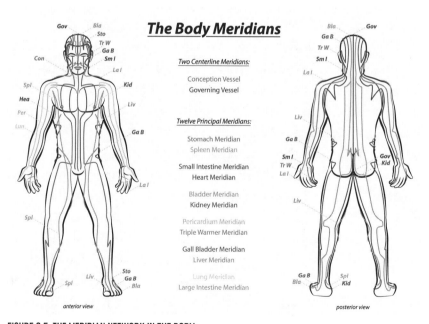

FIGURE 2.5. THE MERIDIAN NETWORK IN THE BODY

It is crucial to understand the concept of meridians in TCM. Meridian channels are the bioelectrical and biochemical energy networks that support good energy *qi* flowing throughout the body. It is akin to the electrical-wiring circuits and the plumbing hidden behind the walls in your house. Your meridian energy network connects organs, tissues, veins, nerves, cells, atoms, and consciousness itself. There are twelve major meridians, each of which connects to one of the twelve major organs—including the teeth, according to TCM theory. Meridians are also related to a variety of phenomena, including circadian rhythms, seasons, and planetary movements, to create additional invisible networks.[71]

Have you heard about the Tooth-Body connection? Each tooth is related to an acupuncture meridian related to various organs, tissues, and glands in the body on this particular meridian or "energy highway." This connection can often indicate your overall health and wellness by reviewing your dental condition. If a person has a weak internal organ, the associated meridian tooth's condition could be considerably more problematic. All the body structures on an individual meridian can be affected when energy flow through that meridian is altered or blocked. Energy flow can be altered in a meridian when an organ on that meridian is diseased or infected.

What does all this mean to you? Well, if you have a bad tooth, the energy flow through the meridian belonging to that tooth will be altered. This, in turn, can affect the health of all the other organs on that meridian. For example, the upper right first molar tooth is on the same meridian as the liver, kidneys, pancreas, stomach, and breast. So, if this tooth has a problem, it may affect energy flow through the meridian, and the health of your liver, kidneys, pancreas, stomach, or breast may be affected as well.

According to Dr. Dawn Ewing, PhD, author of *Let the Tooth Be Known,* 4th edition, a meridian is a giant freeway making a circle around a city. There are several exit and entrance ramps. These ramps allow energy to flow from the meridian to the organ and

Tooth/Organ Connection

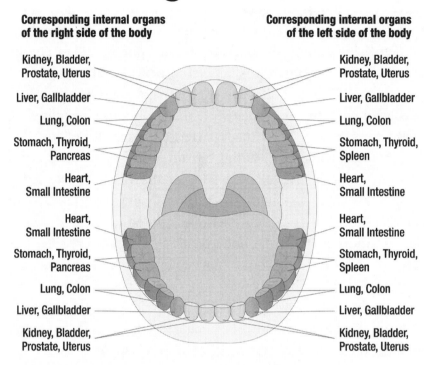

Corresponding internal organs of the right side of the body

Kidney, Bladder, Prostate, Uterus

Liver, Gallbladder

Lung, Colon

Stomach, Thyroid, Pancreas

Heart, Small Intestine

Heart, Small Intestine

Stomach, Thyroid, Pancreas

Lung, Colon

Liver, Gallbladder

Kidney, Bladder, Prostate, Uterus

Corresponding internal organs of the left side of the body

Kidney, Bladder, Prostate, Uterus

Liver, Gallbladder

Lung, Colon

Stomach, Thyroid, Spleen

Heart, Small Intestine

Heart, Small Intestine

Stomach, Thyroid, Spleen

Lung, Colon

Liver, Gallbladder

Kidney, Bladder, Prostate, Uterus

FIGURE 2.6. TOOTH/ORGAN MERIDIAN RELATIONSHIP CHART

from the organ back to the meridian. Imagine knowing it should take an hour to complete one circle on this imaginary freeway, but today, it seems slow. Then imagine sending a helicopter to locate the traffic blockage and report where the blockage is. With this information, you can make choices about what to do. This imaginary scenario happens when you use electrodermal screening – also called a *Meridian Stress Assessment* – to identify the flow of energy and blockages on the meridian pathways.

Meridians are simply the electrical wiring conduits arranged along the main twelve pathways in your body's electrical flow. Just as your car's electrical wiring is logically laid out to power the car's engine, your meridians are logically laid out to power your body from your gut.

Cell Voltage

Let us define the term "voltage." Voltage is the electrical capacity difference between two separate points. In the AA battery, the potential difference is between the top (+) and bottom (−) of the battery cell. The electrical voltage is the result of the excess of negative charge at the negative pole.[23] The functional significance of voltage lies within this potential difference between two separate points in a circuit, where the electrostatic field production follows.

You can witness this phenomenon during thunderstorms. Mother Nature's grand display of an electrostatic field is generated between the clouds in the sky and the earth. When the field becomes too strong,

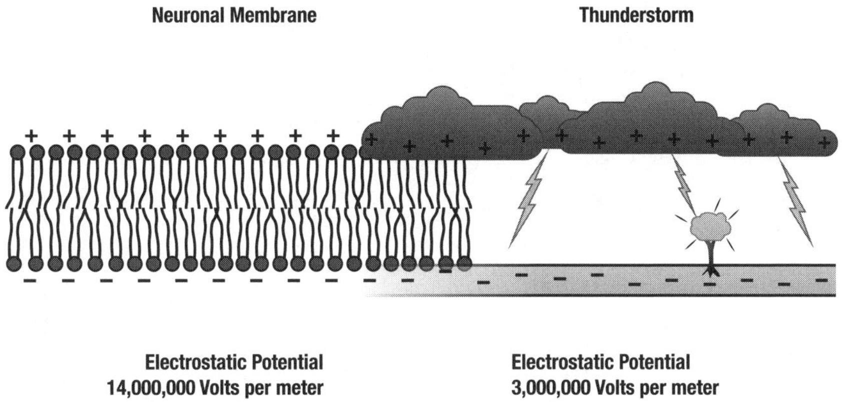

Neuronal Membrane　　　　**Thunderstorm**

Electrostatic Potential
14,000,000 Volts per meter

Electrostatic Potential
3,000,000 Volts per meter

FIGURE 2.7. THE ELECTROSTATIC FIELD COMPARISON

it produces lightning. It is the spark of electricity that shoots the gap between the positive and the negative poles. During lightning storms, the electrostatic field is supercharged to a millionfold. According to energy-field calculations, the strength of a lightning field is about 3 million volts per meter! Such a storm is how Mother Nature recharges the earth with more life-sustaining negative electrons.

In molecular biology, according to Bruce Lipton, PhD, a single cell has a voltage with an electric potential of about −40 to −80 m Volts (0.04 to 0.08 volts) across the cell membranes. 50 trillion cells × .07volts = 3.5 trillion volts. The body's total voltage is equal to 3.5 trillion volts![24]

Let us compare the electrical field phenomenon between your body's electrical charge to the power of a lightning strike. Your body has a total voltage of 3.5 trillion volts, while the lightning strike has only 3 million volts. The only difference is that what occurs inside the cell membrane is a micro event, while the thunderstorm is a macro display. However, it illustrates that your body is a super machine with a massive, bioelectric, super rechargeable battery.

This super machine body must be wired in an organized pathway to hold the 3.5 trillion volts effectively. The twelve meridians are your body's way of organizing this electrical wiring layout. Every single cell must be electrically connected to form tissues via a specific meridian line. They are the invisible electrical lines that carry energy throughout your body.

Some of the most vital elements in our bodies include calcium (Ca++), Sodium (Na+), Potassium (K+), and Chloride (Cl−). The positive or negative ions symbol next to their chemical name signifies their electrical charge. Almost all of our cells can use these charged elements, called *ions*, to generate electricity. The contents of the cell are protected from the outside environment by a cell membrane. The cell membrane acts as a way for the battery to generate electrical currents.[25]

The electrochemical charges of every cell are located in the cell membrane. Charges can be neutral, positive, or negative. Cells must maintain a specific ideal voltage to sustain a healthy biological process. Each cell communicates with those surrounding it via electrochemical signals. Your mitochondria are your power cells that maintain an electrical charge that is critical to your energy production. A standard cell charge is slightly on the negative side, which is −40mV (million Volts), enough to power itself. It must increase higher than −40 mV to regenerate a new cell.[26] When our cell's electrical charge decreases by at least −5mV, fatigue starts to set in. The prolonged, uncorrected, low-cell voltage will reverse the polarity from a negative to a positive charge. This polarity reversal will eventually lead to diseases, damaged DNA, tumor growth, and infections.[27] This is how the disease process begins. Your body begins by giving hints, such as fatigue. The beginning of this process could be triggered simply by dehydration, stress, lack of sleep, or an unhealthy diet. All your epigenetic choices are a direct influence on your body's electrical voltage. You can heal and stay healthy by maintaining an optimal voltage and maintaining your efficient meridian energy flow.[26]

For your body to be in optimal health, it must maintain a consistent electrical charge to efficiently power all the cells. The typical values of a healthy cell membrane electrical voltage are between −40 mV and −80 mV. This electrical charge has two essential functions. First, the cell acts as a battery, supplying power to operate *molecular devices* built in the membrane. Second, it transmits signals between the electrically excitable cells, such as neurons and muscle cells.

Dr. Abraham Liboff, MD, an orthopedic surgeon, has contributed significant research on the use of micro-electrical energy for healing your body. He treated a patient with a non-union (non-healing bone fracture) broken bone, scheduled for amputation because of *pseudoarthrosis*. *Pseudoarthrosis* is the abnormal union formed by fibrous tissue between parts of the bone that was fractured. Dr. Liboff saved the patient's leg by applying microcurrent from a single dry cell to the break between the two disconnected or nonunion bones. As hoped, the bones healed until they were as good as new! It proves the practical application of electrical energy medicine as a healing modality in the body.[28] His findings excited physicists, but, unfortunately, not the medical scientific community.

If you ever studied chemistry, you may remember that all the periodic table molecules show their corresponding electrical charge. Individual biologically charged particles or ions play an essential dynamic role in human physiology. The application of physics principles into biochemical physiology within the body just makes sense. For example, charged particles, like magnesium (Mg) and calcium (Ca), exhibit magnetic, electrical charges within the body. They help maintain the body's electrical load, hence the name *electrolytes*. They contain electrical energy charges. Every food or drink we consume has an electrical charge from its molecular component. Therefore, eating the right food means recharging your body with the proper electrical charge it needs.

Meridian-based Healing Modalities

Many known healing modalities are using the principles of the meridians. An ancient medical system using hair-thin needles to activate or enhance the meridian flow is a form of electrical energy medicine called *acupuncture*. Other modern modalities employ both passive and active electrical stimulation. Examples of these include a practice called "earthing" and macro-, micro-, and even nano-electrical current healing treatments.

Acupuncture

The practice of acupuncture is an effective healing practice performed for thousands of years in Asia. Traditional Chinese Medicine (TCM) was able to map the meridian electrical pathways of the body. Each meridian pathway connects systematically to a corresponding organ, from head to toe. All of our body parts are interconnected. For example, your teeth have corresponding meridians connecting to your organs in your gut, in your spine, and even down to your hands and feet! Acupuncturists found that using hair-thin needles strategically along the twelve meridian pathways will open a blockage and stimulate the flow of the body's electrical wiring back to a healing voltage level.

Besides nutritional medicine, I use acupuncture as part of my holistic physical therapy. I give my patients an option to use acupuncture as an additional healing device. I believe in recharging the voltage before attempting any therapeutic exercise. Your muscle cells need to be in a fully charged electrical energy state to begin the healing process. For some people, acupuncture works right away, but, for most people, it may take several sessions to work, depending on the severity of the voltage deficiency.

Earthing

Earthing, or grounding, is a healthy practice of harvesting the negative electrons from Mother Earth by direct contact with our skin, maybe by walking barefoot on the sand, grass, tile, or concrete. It is simply walking on the bare ground. Earthing is also known as "*vitamin G.*"

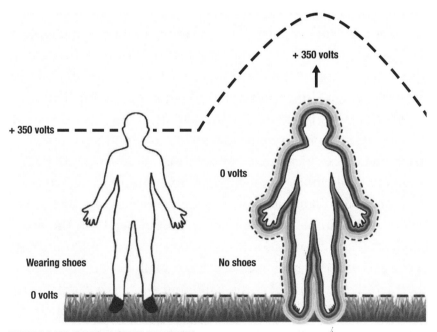

FIGURE 2.8. THE UMBRELLA EFFECT OF EARTHING

As you already know, every cell of your body has negative and positive ions. Typically, our body has a charge of −50 to −80 mV. Any reversal of polarity to the positive charge (+) will almost guarantee the development of disease processes, the damaging DNA, stimulation of tumor growths, and/or an increase in inflammation and likelihood of infection. Once weakened, your body will require more than the −50 to −70 mV to fully regenerate and repair. An increased positive charge (+) will increase inflammation, which will lead to various chronic degenerative diseases. The negative electrons (−), on the other hand, reduce inflammation and promote health.

Having our skin or feet directly in contact with Mother Earth's energy source is the best way to recharge healthy negative electrons into our body. It will surge the body's electrical charge from zero to approximately 350 volts. The concept is that the earth contains a mild negative charge that can restore your body's standard electrical charge. In modern-day living, we have isolated our direct contact with Mother Earth. Every time we use a nonconductive material, such as rubber (in our shoes), plastics, wood, laminate, and asphalt (in flooring surfaces), we prevent ourselves from accessing the natural anti-inflammatory benefits of *earthing*. *Earthing* not only reduces inflammation, it also improves overall physiological function.[28]

There are two types of inflammation: acute and chronic. Acute inflammation is our immune system's natural initial response to injury and illness. Ideally, with a healthy immune system, our body is supposed to manage acute inflammation immediately. You can imagine acute inflammation like a small house fire, put out quickly by our body's immune system, or "extinguisher." On the other hand, chronic inflammation is the unresolved acute inflammation over a prolonged period from a weak or malfunctioning immune system. You can think of chronic inflammation as a raging forest fire. This type of chronic, uncontrolled inflammation is often the initial aggravator that drives most degenerative chronic diseases.

Our body's metabolic byproducts create free radicals, which can be understood as "good guys" turned "bad guys." Once the free radicals have done their clean-up job, our bodies use antioxidants, or negative electrons, like a fire extinguisher, putting out the fire of inflammation. But if we do not have enough negative electrons, the fire or inflammation continues to burn out of control. To get it under control, we need to have an abundant supply of antioxidants, supplying negative electrons. We have an unlimited supply of negative electrons available to us from Mother Earth; just simply connect any of your bare skin to the ground.

In the 1990s, the National Institute of Environmental Health Sciences was compiling a paper on the effects EMFs have on human health. It was the beginning of scientific studies on earthing. It revealed that the practice of earthing has significant physiological benefits and defuses the causes of acute and chronic inflammation. In 2015, an earthing study on inflammation, wound healing, prevention, and treatment of chronic inflammatory and autoimmune diseases found that grounding reduces pain and alters the numbers of circulating neutrophils and lymphocytes in the bloodstream. It also

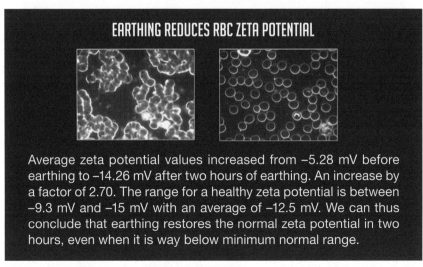

EARTHING REDUCES RBC ZETA POTENTIAL

Average zeta potential values increased from –5.28 mV before earthing to –14.26 mV after two hours of earthing. An increase by a factor of 2.70. The range for a healthy zeta potential is between –9.3 mV and –15 mV with an average of –12.5 mV. We can thus conclude that earthing restores the normal zeta potential in two hours, even when it is way below minimum normal range.

FIGURE 2.9. RED BLOOD CELLS: BEFORE AND AFTER EARTHING

has a positive effect on the chemical factors related to inflammation.[29] Earthing is the best and most efficient way to increase your cellular voltage to prevent or neutralize inflammation without medications.

Earthing is also an effective blood thinner, as investigated in the study entitled, *"Earthing or Grounding the Human Body Reduces Blood Viscosity—a Major Factor in Cardiovascular Disease,"* by Dr. Stephen Sinatra, MD, and colleagues. This study revealed that grounding or earthing has an intriguing effect on human physiology and health, including beneficial effects on various cardiovascular risk factors.[30] This study examined the impact of two hours of grounding on the electrical charge (*zeta potential,* or *the degree of negative charge on the surface of a red blood cell*) on red blood cells (RBCs) and the effect on the extent of RBC clumping of diseased cells. The result of the study revealed that earthing recharged red blood cell function and reversed clumping (see Figure 12). When comparing this remarkable natural healing process with a drug marketed as a blood thinner, it is noteworthy that the drug is technically only blocking your blood from clotting and not actually thinning your blood.

According to a 2014 book by Clinton Ober, *Earthing: The Most Important Health Discovery Ever*, there are myriad physiologic benefits to earthing. It reduces acute and chronic pain, and it improves sleep through coordination of your circadian rhythm with Mother Earth, thus producing the proper hormones to induce sleep.[31] Earthing provides a calming effect on the brain; it improves anxiety, irritability, and depression, influenced by the hormone cortisol.[32] It also increases energy by supercharging your cells to an optimal voltage charge for healing and repair.[33] Since the cells are supercharged, it lowers cell stress. It also lessens hormonal and menstrual symptoms.[34]

Additionally, earthing reduces jetlag by normalizing the body's biorhythms from time zone differences during travel.[30] Earthing promotes a 54 percent reduction of midnight cortisol levels, which leads to better sleep. It also increases the early-morning cortisol production by 34 percent, thus improving daytime energy levels. Earthing can also protect us by neutralizing daily electromagnetic fields, such as excessive mobile phone usage, excessive computer usage, and exposure to low-frequency EMFs, as discussed in Book One.

Modern-day living and modern footwear have reduced our direct contact with Mother Earth's electrical current. The application of rubber soles in contemporary footwear is not conducive to earthing activities, like walking barefoot on the ground. We are consequently prevented from regular access to the bioelectrical healing benefits of Mother Earth.

Clint Ober started the grounding movement. He also discovered indoor grounding products. You can now harvest Mother Earth's therapeutic electrons regularly at night while sleeping. He designed grounding products which you can plug directly into your household electrical outlets.[35] I am grounding myself while writing this book.

THE ENDOCANNABINOID SYSTEM

Most people have not heard about the endocannabinoid system (ECS). The word "endocannabinoid" stems from endogenous (a substance or process originating from within an organism, tissue, or cell) and cannabinoid (named for the plant, cannabis). The terms "endocannabinoid" and "endogenous cannabinoid" refer to the same thing and are used interchangeably.

The endocannabinoid system was discovered in 1964 by an Israeli scientist, Dr. Raphael Mechoulam often called the godfather of cannabinoid research. He was the first to identify cannabidiol (CBD) and then a year later identified and isolated tetrahydrocannabinol (THC). THC is the main psychoactive compound in cannabis that produces a high sensation. Both compounds interact with your body's endocannabinoid system, but they have very different effects.[36]

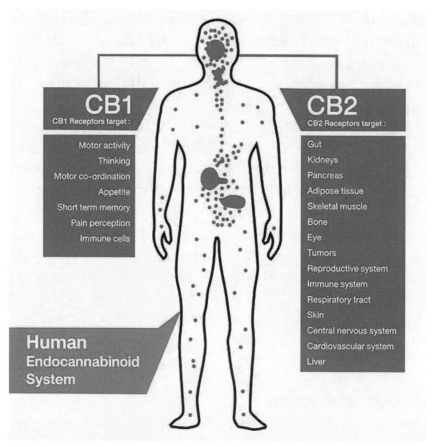

FIGURE 2.10. THE ENDOCANNABINOID SYSTEM

In 1988, Allyn Howlett and William Devane discovered the first cannabinoid receptor in a rat's brain.[37] They began to map the brain's CB receptors and found more of these receptors than any other neurotransmitter receptor.[38]

The endocannabinoid system is a fantastic system that regulates our body's remarkable network of endocannabinoids and cannabinoid receptors that exist throughout our body. Cannabinoid receptors exist on the surface of cells and "listen" to what is going on in the body. They communicate this information about our bodies' status and changing circumstances to the inside of the cell, allowing for the appropriate action. In other words, they help us maintain homeostasis by monitoring what is going on in our bodies.

Initially, research suggested endocannabinoid receptors were only present in the brain and nerves. Scientists later found that the receptors are present throughout the body, including our skin, immune cells, bone, fat tissue, liver, pancreas, skeletal muscle, heart, blood vessels, kidney, and gastrointestinal tract.[39]

The endocannabinoid system (ECS) is a complex cell-signaling system. The ECS involves three core components: endocannabinoids, receptors, and enzymes. Endocannabinoids, also called endogenous cannabinoids, are molecules made by your body. They are functionally similar to plant-based cannabinoids, but your body produces them.[40]

Experts have identified two key endocannabinoids so far: anandamide (AEA) and 2-arachidonoylglyerol (2-AG). These endocannabinoids help keep internal functions running smoothly. Your body produces them as needed, making it difficult to know what typical levels are for each.[41]

Endocannabinoid receptors are found throughout your body. Endocannabinoids bind to them to signal that the ECS needs to act. There are two primary endocannabinoid receptors: CB1 receptors, mostly found in the central nervous system, CB2 receptors, mostly found in your peripheral nervous system, especially immune cells. Endocannabinoids can bind to either receptor. The effects that result depend on where the receptor is located and which endocannabinoid it binds to. For example, endocannabinoids might target CB1 receptors in a spinal nerve to relieve pain. Others might bind to a CB2 receptor in your immune cells to signal that your body's experiencing inflammation, a common sign of autoimmune disorders.[42]

Through CB1 and CB2 receptors, the ECS helps regulate a lot of essential functions, such as appetite and digestion, metabolism, immune function, chronic pain, inflammation, mood, sleep, reproduction/fertility, motor control, temperature regulation, memory and learning, cardiovascular functioning, muscle formation, bone health, liver function, pleasure/reward, stress, and skin and nerve function.[38]

The third component of ECS is the enzymes. ECS enzymes are responsible for breaking down endocannabinoids once they have carried out their function. There are two main enzymes responsible for this: fatty acid amide hydrolase, which breaks down AEA; monoacylglycerol acid lipase, which typically breaks down 2-AG.[40]

Some experts believe in a theory known as *Clinical Endocannabinoid Deficiency* (CECD). This theory suggests that low endocannabinoid levels in your body or ECS dysfunction can contribute to the development of certain conditions. A 2016 study reviewed over ten years of research on the subject, and the researchers suggested an ECS connection for why some people develop migraines, fibromyalgia, and irritable bowel syndrome.[43] None of these conditions have an exact underlying cause. They are also often resistant to treatment and sometimes occur alongside each other.[44]

If CECD does play any role in these conditions, targeting the ECS or endocannabinoid production could be the missing key to treatment, but more research is needed. The bottom line is that ECS plays a significant role in keeping your internal processes stable. But there is still a lot we do not know about it. As experts develop a better understanding of the ECS, it could eventually hold the key to treating several conditions.

THE LYMPHATIC SYSTEM

The lymphatic system is known as the *protect-and-transport* system or the *detox-and-defense* system. According to Webster's dictionary, the lymphatic system is that part of the circulatory system concerned, especially, with scavenging fluids and proteins that have escaped

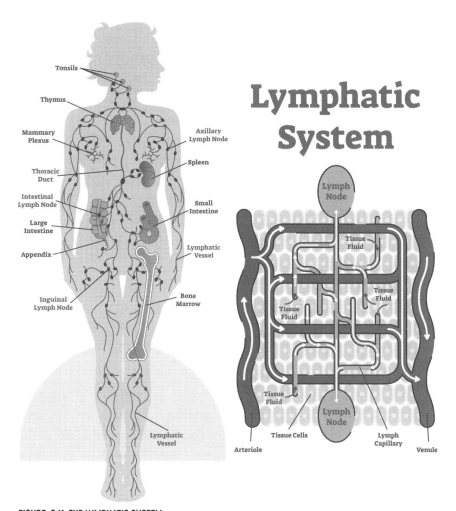

FIGURE. 2.11. THE LYMPHATIC SYSTEM

from cells and tissues and return them to the blood. It runs along with the venous circulatory system. The lymphatic system is the central plumbing for the immune system to remove and destroy waste, debris, dead blood cells, pathogens, toxins, and cancer cells. It is also your vitamins' main delivery transport to your cells. Your lymphatic system's principal assets are water, healthy fats, and some proteins.

Here is how it works:

The lymphatic system is the network of vessels through which lymph drains from the tissues into the blood. Lymph is a colorless fluid containing white blood cells that bathes the tissues and drains through the lymphatic system into the bloodstream. The extensive lymphatic system connects the lymph nodes in the body to each other and the bloodstream. The lymph fluid is the colorless fluid in the lymphatic vessels. It originates from the plasma, the fluid portion of the blood. As the arterial blood rushes out from the heart, it slows down around the small capillary beds. It is this slowing down that allows the plasma to be squeezed out from the blood tissues. It becomes tissue fluid and drains into the lymphatic system.

After the lymph leaves the tissues, the lymph must enter a massive network of specialized lymphatic plumbing systems or capillaries. It has two central network locations: 70 percent of the superficial network vessels or "plumbing" parts are located near or just one millimeter under your skin; the remaining 30 percent are the deep lymphatic capillaries or plumbing surrounding most of the organs. It functions for systematic access during the easy cell cleanup, your body's effective defense with white blood cells (WBC), and for an efficient delivery system of fat-soluble nutrients used by the cells.

Your bone marrow produces antibodies and WBC. It stores them in your blood and lymph tissues. Because white blood cells have a short life of one-to-three days, your bone marrow is always making them. Lymphocytes make up roughly 20 to 40 percent of the total number of cells in the blood and lymph. They are made in your bone marrow and thymus gland. Your WBCs are your protective cell army for fighting invading bacteria, viruses, and other microbial invaders.

The lymphatic system must consistently drain its lymph fluids on a one-way journey from the spaces between cells upward toward the base of either side of the neck, via your subclavian veins, to prevent water clogging in tissues and cells. As lymph fluids move upward toward the neck, the lymph passes through lymph nodes, which filter it to remove debris and pathogens. Besides, it gathers the cleaned lymph fluid and returns it to your bloodstream to maintain overall fluid balance. Since the lymphatic system does not have the heart to pump it, its upward movement

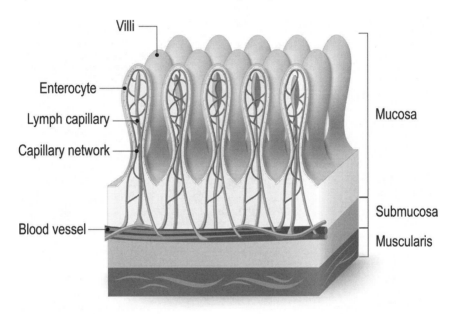

FIGURE 2.12. THE CROSS-SECTION OF THE INTESTINAL WALL AND A SINGLE VILLUS SHOWING THE CAPILLARY AND LYMPHATIC SUPPLY

depends on the muscle and joint pumps' motions. The lymphatic system will get activated by the milking and pumping action of the musculoskeletal movements against gravity. It is the first system that will slow down during inactivity and prolonged bed rest.[45]

There is an essential connection between your gut and your lymphatic system. The lymphatic system absorbs fats and fat-soluble vitamins from your stomach and delivers these nutrients to the body cells, where they are used by your cells. Take note: 80 percent of your vitamins are fat-soluble.

Let us start in your gut lining, specifically your *lacteal duct*. Your lacteal duct never gets any credit for its significant role in your health. Your lacteal duct is an essential unit strategically located on the surface of your gut lining. After digestion, the primary macronutrients are broken down into their essential molecules, for

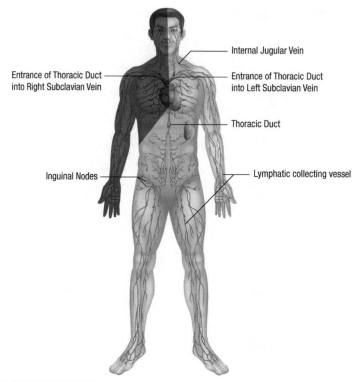

FIGURE 2.13. THE TWO LYMPHATIC PATHWAYS

example, carbohydrates into glucose, fats into essential fatty acids and ketones and omega fats and proteins into amino acids, and so forth. Your lacteal duct's primary function is to absorb good fats, like essential fatty acids and ketones, directly from your gut. It then carries and delivers the absorbed essential fatty acids directly to your heart's main left ventricle, via your left subclavian vein, as well as to your brain. You have a unique plumbing system in your body that is solely for fat transport. That is how vital fat is in your body function.

There are two main lymphatic drainage pathways in your body: the right and the left subclavian veins (see Figure 2.13). Think of them as two drainage and plumbing rivers: the first is for biological sewage, and the second is for nutrient delivery system inside your body. The primary lymphatic path, which includes your left arm, your left upper trunk, your lower chest, and your legs, drains into the left subclavian vein. The second smaller lymphatic pathway, located in your right arm and your right upper trunk, drains into the right subclavian vein.

The next component to be familiar with is your lymph nodes. There is an extensive network of lymph nodes strategically located throughout our bodies. Lymph nodes are significant small structures designed to filter harmful substances, like foreign particles and cancer cells. Most of our immune cells can help fight infection by attacking and destroying germs carried through the lymph fluid. They function as security checkpoints that stop, neutralize, and attack, if necessary, any foreign microbial invaders in your body. When you can feel the hardening of your lymph nodes, it means that there is an ongoing battle in those sites. Your body is busy neutralizing microbial threats in the surrounding territory. For example, if you can feel hardening in your lymph node in the right groin, your body could be fighting inflammation from a microbial threat around the right leg. With a healthy lymphatic system, microbial threats usually resolve themselves without additional help.

Lymph nodes play a significant role in the fight against cancer cells. They are our first line of defense. Premature removal of our lymph nodes during the critical early stage of cancer maybe not a good idea. In 2010, a randomized study by the International Breast Cancer Study Group was done. This study included 934 breast cancer patients from twenty-seven centers in Europe, South America, and Australia. The investigators found significant evidence to support the current practice of not performing an axillary dissection when the tumor burden in the sentinel nodes is minimal or moderate in patients with early onset of breast cancer.[46] Instead, we should boost our lymphatic system with a proper diet and proper lymphatic treatment interventions.

Finally, your lymphoid organs include the thymus, the spleen, the bone marrow, the lymph nodes, and the mucosa-associated lymphoid tissue in your gut, lungs, reproductive organs, and urinary organs. These are the main permanent structures where the migratory immune cells produce, mature, and interact with antigens. Think of antigens as the "bad guys," the foreign microbial invaders that attack the cells inside your body. The thymus and bone marrow are considered the primary lymphatic organs because they are the factories for the "soldier cells": "B" and "T" cells. These cells are programmed in the thymus to distinguish between self and nonself. They are programmed to attack only foreign invaders and not the body tissues.

Secondary lymphoid organs include lymph nodes and the spleen, which filter lymph and blood, respectively, and where naïve B and T cells are introduced to antigens. The antigen is a toxin or other foreign substance that induces an immune response in the body, namely, antibodies' production.

The third lymphatic tissues and organs are the Peyer's patches and surface-associated lymphoid group. They are permanent protective lymphatic stations strategically located on the surface of your lungs and in your gut. They have fancy medical names according to their location; in the lungs, they are known as the *Bronchial-Associated Lymphoid Tissue* (BALT); in your stomach, they are known as the *Gut-Associated Lymphoid Tissue* (GALT). These two locations are where our immune system is regulated. Immunologic-resistance functions happen by memory and by effector cells. In the immune system, effector cells are the relatively short-lived, activated cells that defend the body in an immune response. Effector B cells are called plasma cells and secrete antibodies, and activated T cells include cytotoxic T cells and helper T cells, which carry out cell-mediated responses.[47] Immunological memory is the immune system's ability to quickly and specifically recognize an antigen that the body has previously encountered and has initiated a corresponding immune response against.[48]

Your lymphatic system is also the body's primary amino acids (digested protein) transport system. The size of the protein molecule matters; the smaller the molecule, the better the lymphatic flow. It is important to note a significant difference in protein molecules' size between plant-based proteins and animal-based proteins. Animal-based proteins, such as casein, have bigger particles compared to plant-based proteins. There is even a difference in casein particle size among the animal-based proteins. Both sheep's milk and goat's milk are closer to human milk than cow's milk. Goat's milk is almost identical to breast milk, so babies who cannot tolerate cow's milk may do quite well on goat's milk. A 2018 study was conducted on the structural comparison of casein in cow's milk, goat's milk, and sheep's milk, using X-ray scattering. The study found differences in the size and the density of larger-scale protein structures, although, at an atomic level, the kinds of milk protein—structural configuration was similar.[49]

The interchange gate between the blood vessel and the lymphatic valve is very delicate. It prefers a smaller-size protein molecule. This may be the reason why plant-based protein is more readily absorbable than animal-based protein. As it is sized in casein, animal-based protein may clog the entrance into our lymphatic system. Consequently, a person gets sick; however, lots of soup without animal-based protein helps the lymphatic flow and speeds up recovery.

Unfortunately, our lymphatic system is not well appreciated and is not given enough importance in its massive role in our health and healing. Western medicine undervalues its position, especially in surgical techniques. It is commonly ignored and butchered during surgeries, especially around the abdominal area. The injury or surgical scar's location may eventually block the lymphatic and the meridian electrical flow in the body.[50] Its side effect is subtle initially, but it can be devastating over time as the blockage increases. It may take a few years before you will experience the full adverse effects of lymphatic and bioelectrical obstruction from scar tissues.

Another factor in lymphatic blockage is constant physical compression. Tight garments, especially bras, impinge on the strategic lymphatic organ locations. For women, underwire bras or tight clothing place constant pressure on the breasts, where significant lymphatic drainage areas are located. Your axillary area, also known as your armpit, has direct access to the grand central station for all your upper-body nerves and blood circulation. This grand central station is called the brachial plexus. It is also where major lymphatic plumbing and central lymphatic nodes are located. Topical application of aluminum is a very toxic habit. It is one of the most common ingredients in antiperspirants that work by plugging sweat ducts to stop sweating. Lifetime exposure to toxic aluminum in deodorant leaves you susceptible to aluminum in your bloodstream via sweat glands and skin pores in your armpit. Eventually, the aluminum may breach the protection of the armpit lymph nodes. Once this happens, your body becomes vulnerable to disease and even cancer.

Aluminum can cause genetic mutations, which increases the chances of tumor growth.[51] In a 2014 study, the investigators summarized the possible correlation between heavy metals, epigenetics alterations, and brain tumors.[52] It is found that the presence of aluminum in your system is also linked to cancer and reproductive toxicity.[53] Besides, other deodorant ingredients are known to disrupt our endocrine system. They include triclosan, parabens, phthalates, fragrance, diethanolamine, butane, and isobutane. Minimizing exposure to these harmful chemicals in your hygiene and cosmetic products is a simple way to be a good steward of your health.

Recently, researchers have also found a lymphatic system in the brain, called the *glymphatic system.*[54] Besides waste elimination, the glymphatic system also functions to distribute non-waste compounds, such as glucose, lipids, amino acids, and neurotransmitters, related to volume transmission, into the brain. It detoxifies and restores the brain during deep sleep. More on sleep in Book Three.

Human touch is the primary healing modality of the lymphatic system because of its location. Your superficial lymphatic plumbing system is strategically situated a few millimeters under your skin, which is why human touch is so effective. It is where your WBCs travel. The lymphatic system is your body's protection and defense against infection. Touch activates the increased flow of the lymphatic system—making touch is incredibly healing. A loving and kind touch from another person raises the healing effect exponentially. Touch can also infuse healing energy from another human being. Figuratively speaking, therapeutic massages are like taking 1,000 vitamins because they prime the lymphatic system, improve lymphatic flow, induce increased immune system function, and promote relaxation.

There are many easy and effective methods to improve your lymphatic system. First, proper hydration is fundamentally essential. It is the simplest and most effective start in improving your health. Proper hydration will be a recurring theme in this book, and its importance cannot be over-emphasized. The amount of filtered water you need to drink daily is at least half of your body weight equal in ounces, with a pinch of ancient sea salt per ounce. For example, if you weigh 150 pounds, you need to drink at least seventy-five ounces of filtered water daily. It should be mildly saline or mildly alkaline water because the salt aids the water molecule to enter your cell membrane.

Besides, plenty of restorative sleep, as well as regular exercise daily, both cardio training and strength training, are important ways to improve your lymphatic system dramatically. A healthy diet that includes good fats is vital. I also highly recommend getting a regular massage to keep the lymphatic fluids flowing. Many people also benefit from manual lymph drainage therapy. Finally, shake it up with whole-body gravity-resisted vibration and rebounding therapies. These are great lymphatic modalities to diversify your healing practices and improve your overall wellbeing.

I experienced the compelling power of manual lymphatic therapy while growing up. I grew up with the ancient Filipino art of healing. The practitioners are called a *manghihilot* (a *hilot* practitioner) and an albularyo (an herbalist). Hilot is a hands-on healing art that involves the body-mind connection and deep-tissue massage. The *manghihilot* intuitively scan the body with the hand, touching the pulse on your wrist to diagnose energetically imbalanced areas.[55] The *manghihilot* can focus on the affected area to work from this energy-field scan information and give balance and relief.

When I was ten years old, I severely twisted and fractured my right wrist from falling out of a mango tree. My mother immediately took me across the Layawan River by boat to see the town's *manghihilot* lady. I remember walking into a dark bamboo hut set upon shaky stilts and filled with the scent of incense. She was a mystical, very old, wrinkled lady, to my ten-year-old eyes. She was whispering a prayer and proceeded to manipulate my elbow to align it manually. It was a harrowing experience. I clearly remembered the different herbs' intense aroma with coconut oil wrapped in banana leaves around my right wrist and forearm (an herbal poultice). I had to wear the homemade herb pack wrapped in banana leaves daily. After three weeks, we returned to see her; my right wrist had healed. My wrist function was fully restored, pain-free! This ancient art of *hilot* is incredibly effective. There should be more studies on *hilot* and *albularyo* to integrate them into mainstream healing modalities. We may learn a great deal and incorporate these ancient pearls of wisdom in modern medicine.

THE DIGESTIVE SYSTEM

In my PT studies, I was not taught that 80 percent of my immune cells were located in my digestive system. The digestive system is the primary defense against external invaders that enter your stomach through your mouth. The intestinal lining is protected with mucus to defend against microbes and foreign substances. Your digestive system contains approximately 25 to 30 feet of muscular hose that runs from the mouth to the anus. It is in a north-to-south orientation, meaning that the flow starts from the top, with your mouth, and goes down to your anus. Your digestive system works most efficiently when it is in an upright orientation because gravity significantly helps with the downward flow from the start to the endpoint. So, sit up in the chair or on the floor when eating, no lying down.

After eating, walking also helps your digestion function better. This is because your legs are connected to your hips, pelvic muscles, and abdominal muscles, where your gut is housed. The walking helps pull and push the abdominal muscles, which are also connected to your intestinal muscles. Walking, therefore, dramatically helps with digestive contractions.

In the next chapter, you will learn in detail about your gut's digestion basics.

 Your self-healing system: autonomic nervous system, meridians, endocannabinoid system, lymphatic system, and digestive system.

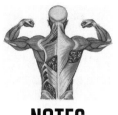

NOTES

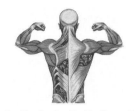

CHAPTER 7

YOUR GUT: YOUR BODY'S ENGINE

"All health and diseases begin in the gut."
—Hippocrates

In this chapter, I will discuss in detail the incredible way in which your digestive system works and operates. This foundational knowledge of your gut will significantly aid you in facilitating the epigenetic mechanism of efficient digestion. Nurturing gut health feeds the mind and the entire body.

YOUR BODY'S ENGINE: DIGESTION 101

The foods that you select, cook, serve, and eat influence the effectiveness of your digestion. The right raw materials and subsequent proper digestion allow your body to absorb the essential nutrients and put them to work. Digestion consumes approximately 70 to 80 percent of your metabolic energy. Your stomach uses most of your blood during digestion, and, if necessary, it will even borrow blood from your brain. It is the reason why you get sleepy after a big meal; your heart, brain, and muscles lend blood to the gut for digestion. This is also the main reason you should not exercise intensely after eating.

If, for example, you have a weak heart, exercising after eating may cause a sudden massive heart attack because of a dramatic decrease in blood circulation in the heart after meals.

The Digestive Process

Optimal health requires the synergistic coordination of the three digestive processes. They are as follows: mechanical coordination, biochemical coordination, and bacterial coordination. The mechanical function is the chewing function of the teeth, the jaw, and the saliva to break down food into micro-digestible particles. Ideally, it is suggested that you chew the food at least twenty to thirty times, almost converting it into liquid form before you swallow it. With the food at a nearly fluid state, your mouth can break down many of the carbohydrates and extract the enzymes. Starchy food will get predigested by salivary enzymes in the mouth. Saliva contains a substance called *Epidermal Growth Factor* (EGF) produced only in the salivary glands. EGF is a potent stimulator of cell growth in the liver. Chewing food thoroughly will encourage EGF production. Many documented cases of chronically ill patients have shown dramatic improvement only by adequately chewing their food.[56]

The next process is the biochemical digestion phase. Your stomach produces and uses your stomach acids, called hydrochloric acid, to biochemically breakdown the liquid food bolus from your mouth. After all, your stomach does not have teeth! So, when food is poorly chewed in the mouth, the stomach must compensate by increasing stomach acid's biochemical production. Stomach acids' primary functions are to disinfect and break down the food into micro-absorbable sizes. When food is poorly chewed, it will require double or triple the amount of stomach acids. The additional acids will eventually wear down the stomach lining and slow the digestive process. More on stomach acids will appear in the next section.

The third process of digestion is a bacterial function. Our digestive system must maintain the ideal balance of good versus harmful bacteria. The ratio should be roughly 80 percent of good bacteria to 20 percent of harmful bacteria. This balance will be threatened if your diet is high in sugar and carbohydrates. Excessive sugar and carbohydrate consumption cause harmful bacteria to grow uncontrollably, overwhelm, and eventually kill the good bacteria. Bacteria eat what we eat. Sugar feeds harmful bacteria. For example, *H. pylori* is a bacterium that usually lives in the gut and kept in check to a healthy minimum level. Foods that are high in sugar and carbohydrates stimulate *H. pylori*'s overpopulation, which turns it into an overpopulation of harmful bacteria. This usually leads to serious gut issues. Good bacteria, or *probiotics*, are fed on *prebiotics*, which are vegetable fibers and fermented vegetables.

Bacterial digestive action also produces most of our vitamins in the small intestines. Therefore, your gut microbiota is critical to your overall health. Gut microbes have the power to heal and protect your brain, your immune function, your mental performance, your emotional stability, and the internal regulation of the body's inflammatory tendency. More on microbiota will be covered in Chapter 8 of this book.

Digestion and Stomach Acids

The term "acids" might have a negative connotation, but do not worry. God made your stomach acids super healthy for a good reason. Stomach acids are actually healthy and were created with great design. As mentioned above, your stomach acids are the first line of your biochemical protection from harmful microorganisms that invade the body via food. The stronger your stomach acids, the better fortified your immune system is, and the better your digestion. Stomach acids are your biggest ally.

Let us go back to our elementary chemistry lessons to review the basics of acidity and alkalinity. Do you remember the pH scale value? pH is the potential hydrogen in a substance. The pH is, in other words, the voltage or electrical charge in a liquid. There is a positive (+) charge electron and a negative (−) charge electron. Scientists use the pH scale measurement ranges from 0–14, where 0–7 is acidic, an electron taker. The pH value 7 is neutral. The pH value ranges from 7–14 is alkaline, an electron donor. Your body has an innate intelligent design that knows when specific chemical pH charges are needed at their respective body parts. It is designed to be a master modulator of your body's ideal pH charge.

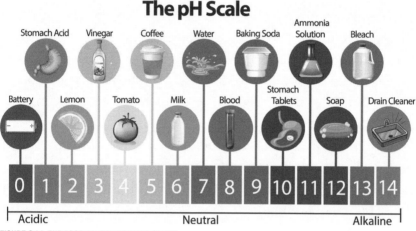

FIGURE 2.14. THE FOOD PH COMPARISON CHART

Your body prefers your nutrition to be in a neutral range, between acidic and alkaline. Any food or beverage with a charge on either end of the pH scale is never good for the body. Healthy vegetables, healthy nuts, and wholesome fats almost always carry a neutral pH score. High-sugar foods and highly processed foods possess very acidic values. You may note in the table above (Figure 2.14) that most house cleansers fall on the alkaline end on the other end of the spectrum. Their primary function is to neutralize the acids, which is the charge of most dirt and grime.

It is critical to note that your stomach acids need to be consistently very acidic at a range of 1 to 3 pH to break down food, especially iron and proteins. This very acidic pH is important for the digestion of both macronutrients and micronutrients. It is how they are broken down into their essential, necessary components and absorbed into the bloodstream for cell use.

Preventive medicine specialist Dr. Jonathan Wright, MD, ND, states in his book *Why Stomach Acid Is Good for You*, "*When your gut is healthy, it will produce a normal stomach acid pH of between 1.5 to 3.0.*" When we talk about stomach acid, it is about the hydrochloric acid (HCl) secreted by your stomach, which has an initial pH value of 0.8. It is purely acid! Imagine if you put your whole fist into a gut with healthy stomach acids. The stomach acids would melt your entire fist, bones, and muscles into a liquid state within five to ten minutes. Your stomach acids must be robust for your body to effectively break down your food into its essential components for efficient absorption. We need to be aware of the crucial functions of strong stomach acids. Unfortunately, this essential information and its pivotal role are severely downplayed in the medical world.

In recent times, food-poisoning cases are increasing in the United States every year because most Americans are developing weak stomach acids from unnecessary and prolonged use of medications, especially antacid, OTC, or prescribed drugs. The steady intake of highly processed food also weakens the system of many Americans. Besides, the unnecessary use of antimicrobial products is killing good bacteria and neutralizing stomach acids. One of the biggest challenges faced by food-borne bacteria is acid. Acidic conditions, particularly in the stomach, will kill most microbes found in contaminated food.[57]

According to Nobel laureate Dr. Otto Warburg, MD, and medical research specialists Sagen Ishizuk, PhD, Kurt Donsbach, DC, ND, PhD, and Sam Graci,

"There is no known disease-causing organism (bacteria, virus, Plasmodium, fungus, yeast, ECT) or degenerative disease

(osteoporosis, arthritis, fibromyalgia, "old age" disease, etc.) that can continue to reproduce or create degeneration in an alkaline-oxygenated environment."[58]

These brilliant doctors have established how to optimize human health by maintaining an ideal alkaline state within the body. When you have healthy stomach acids, harmful microbes cannot invade. At the same time, your stomach acids help your body replenish, regenerate, and repair when given the proper environment and raw materials, which are found chemically in slightly alkaline-charged foods and beverages. Unprocessed foods such as filtered water, properly prepared fresh, organic whole, green vegetables, fruits, and raw nuts are the basics for foundational nutrition that stays within the optimal pH value that your body requires.

A 2008 study showed that the lower the stomach acid pH (more acidic) is, the much lower levels of ingested bacterial pathogens survive in the stomach.[59] The study investigated the crucial role of stomach acids and the effects of hypochlorhydria (low stomach acid pH) on susceptibility to infection. We could apply this study to the food-poisoning cruise scenario; passengers eat the same food while in the boat, but not everybody gets sick. Imagine that 30 percent of the passengers on the cruise got food poisoning while the other 70 percent did not. Suppose you could examine the difference in stomach acid strength between the passengers. In that case, we can surmise that those passengers who have weak stomach acids and who take a constant antacid for digestion will more likely be the ones who suffered from food poisoning. It is crucial to maintain strong hydrochloric acid throughout your lifetime, especially when traveling.

As mentioned previously, your stomach acids maintain the balance in your microbiota of the toxic bacteria and the good bacteria in the stomach. There are trillions of bacteria, viruses, and fungi that live inside and outside of us. Maintaining a properly balanced relationship with them keeps us healthy.

Stomach acids activate the digestive enzymes necessary for macronutrient digestion and absorption. Digestive enzymes are chemical messengers in your gut. Each digestive messenger has its specific territory to alert and bring information to help your digestion. In a healthy gut, digestive enzymes are mobilized only when you have strong stomach acids. You need digestive enzymes, like pepsin, to digest proteins. At the same time, *gastrin* alerts the pancreas to release bicarbonate and pancreatic juices, as the stomach lowers the pH from seven to one, into a very acidic state. In the first segment of the small intestines, the duodenum, cholecystokinin (CCK) is produced and mixed with the digested food to produce *chyme*. Chyme is a semiliquid mass of partially digested food that passes from the stomach through the pyloric sphincter into the duodenum. CCK is a peptide (a group of amino acids from proteins) hormone responsible for stimulating fat and protein digestion. The *chyme* will travel down toward the small intestines, which produce sodium bicarbonate needed to raise the pH to seven, returning the *chyme* to a neutral or alkaline level so it will not burn your small intestines. The chyme then helps the digested carbohydrates and proteins to pass through. In the meantime, the gall bladder releases bile to break down the fats into essential fatty acids.

CCK also acts as a hunger suppressant and helps your stomach feel full or satiated. It is also a neuropeptide activator for the neurons in our brain, part of the central nervous system. The presence of fatty acids and specific amino acids in the chyme enters the duodenum stimulates CCK release. Without the strong stomach acid, to begin with, CCK production will be hampered, too.

The cascading negative consequences of weak stomach acids are extremely damaging to one's health. Your stomach acids have a significant physiological role in digestion, satiety, and anxiety. In other words, it has a direct impact on nutrient absorption, feeling full, and feeling happy.

Most macronutrients must be digested down to their primary molecules and converted into usable nutrients for the body. For example, proteins are a fat-soluble macronutrient, whether plant-based or animal-based. Proteins need healthy levels of hydrochloric acid to break down into essential amino acids. Fats are another macronutrient that needs strong stomach acids to turn them into fatty acids before your body can use them. Carbohydrates also need healthy stomach acid to break down into glucose.

Do you remember a TV commercial that showed a happy man on a jet ski, popping the "purple pill" after overeating hotdogs? That and other antacid advertisements have been wildly convincing. A marketing survey in 2003 has shown that approximately one-half of American adults have used antacids. Twenty-seven percent of adults take two or more doses per month. Seventy-five percent of total antacid consumption is by "heavy users," defined as taking more than six doses per week (statistically less than 5 percent of American adults).[60] By 2008, according to a drug topics article by Dana K. Cassell, acid indigestion and heartburn have plagued about a third of the U.S. population. About 100 million Americans experience heartburn every month. About 15 million battle it at least once a day.[61] Sadly, proprietary antacids represent a multimillion-dollar business in this country. In 2008 alone, antacid sales topped $10 billion annually. This over-usage of antacids is a massive health crisis!

An antacid's main job is to reduce acid in your stomach. Consequently, long-term use of antacids will weaken the production of healthy, strong stomach acids. Imagine the myriad of issues chronically weak stomach acids may yield. One major issue would be nutritional deficiencies since the inability to digest proteins will leave the undigested proteins to decompose and rot in your stomach. Undigested fats become rancid after a while in your stomach, and undigested carbohydrates will ferment in your gut as well. All these undigested macronutrients will cause bloating and wreak havoc on your gut. A lack of strong stomach acids is devastating to your health.

Let me explain why *hyperacidity* or *"acid reflux"* is such a misnomer. It is actually caused by *weak* stomach acids or *not enough* stomach acids for proper digestion. In a stomach with weak acids, the food will not be fully digested ten minutes after eating. It will ferment in the stomach. This fermented food will eventually backflow or *reflux* and bubble up to your food pipe, your esophagus. There, it can eat away or burn the mucosal lining of your throat. At this stage, you will start to feel the heartburn sensation behind the breastbone. Your esophageal lining is not designed to be exposed to undigested fermented, very acidic food. Over time, frequent heartburn can lead to GERD—gastroesophageal reflux disease.

It is not therapeutically wise to be taking OTC antacids or the *purple pill* when you start to experience heartburn symptoms. Antacids are a band-aid that masks the real problem in your gut. Heartburn is a desperate cry for help from your gut to improve your stomach acid's quality, ASAP! If you must use antacids, they should be used only for a short period, not as a regular after-meal habit. If your symptoms persist, seek medical attention, and contact your integrative health care practitioner for further interventions on this matter. Otherwise, it will have a negative long-term consequence on your health because it will handcuff your stomach acids, gradually eating away at your gut.

The micronutrient calcium is a fat-soluble micronutrient. It needs to be broken down with a strong hydrochloric acid (stomach acid) before it can be processed into the blood via vitamin D3 and into the bones via vitamin K2. Long-term use of antacids blocks the absorption of calcium in your stomach, increasing the incidence of osteoporosis or osteopenia.

Moreover, long-term use of antacids will deplete magnesium, which is crucial for bone health, muscle relaxation, and especially the heart muscle's rhythm. Magnesium relaxes the heart muscle, while calcium contracts the heart muscle. Magnesium deficiency or imbalance can affect several of your body's systems. Many people are unaware of the fundamental role it plays in your health. Long-term studies on the impact of high magnesium and fiber diets have shown corresponding potential benefits in cardiovascular health, insulin resistance, hypertension, and chronic muscular and neurological systems' chronic symptoms.

You cannot merely overeat unhealthy foods and then just take a pill with stomach-acid-blocking drugs, believing it will fix the problem without serious side effects. If you have recurring bloating symptoms, please listen to your gut. It is essential to listen to your gut to know when you are satiated as not to overeat. A healthy diet will support your hydrochloric acid production, which will strengthen your digestion overall. I used to suffer from bloating and frequent heartburn pains with migraines after meals. After a visit to the emergency room with severe stomach pains following a Mexican meal, I was diagnosed with acid reflux and moderate GERD. Today, I am free of GERD symptoms because I manage them by chewing my food until it is a liquid consistency and regularly taking supplements. I take a hydrochloric acid supplement prescribed by my naturopath doctor (ND) every day before meals to help with my digestion. I had to change my diet and increase my water consumption thirty minutes before and after meals. I refrain from drinking water while I am eating so that I do not neutralize my stomach acids. More on the proper timing of drinking water can be found in Chapter 11 of Book Three.

DIGESTION AND THE SENSES

Let us start with the upright orientation of our digestion. The functional forward flow starts from north to south or top to bottom.

Our digestion begins from the northern-most end of our body, from our brains through our eyes and nose. Just merely looking at appealing food, whether in person or a photo, triggers the brain to secrete digestive enzymes. The expression that your eyes are bigger than your stomach has a scientific basis. Beautiful, delicious food presentations and different food colors on display activate your brain—the more variety and richness, real or in a photo, the more your mind is stimulated. I believe that God designed food appeal in this way because when we consume an array of naturally colorful foods, we obtain the nutrients our body needs. Colors are our clues to healthy food, even when we do not necessarily know their actual nutritional value.

How should food look? We eat with our eyes first—food presentation matters. When we were hunters and gatherers, Mother Nature gave us vivid cues about which plants and berries were ready to eat. The berries and fruits' color gave an observable hint as to what kind of nutrients, vitamins, and antioxidants the plant possessed. Today, too, your eyes pick up visual cues from food and activate your brain to produce insulin and other necessary digestive enzymes to prepare the food to be eaten.

The next sensory radar for digestion is the olfactory sense—that is, our sense of smell. Good smells usually accompany good-tasting foods that activate the olfactory nerve in the brain and stimulate saliva production in the mouth. The olfactory sense also induces the body to start producing insulin in the blood in anticipation of the food before it arrives in the stomach.

The sense of smell is our most acute sense and most strongly linked to our tastes, memories, and feelings. It has a direct pathway to the brain. Essentially, when you smell something familiar, the memory recall is almost automatic because of the short and direct path to the brain's long-term memory cortex, the hippocampus. When we sniff, odor molecules are drawn in through our nose. The particles then dissolve and penetrate through our nose's mucus membrane. Once inside our nose, it binds with the nose cilia, the hairlike projective receptor cells, and converts the now-dissolved odor molecule into a message or an impulse to the brain via the olfactory nerve. The signals are processed and passed onto other parts of the brain, like the memory and the cortex, which process emotion. When you get a whiff of a familiar perfume fragrance, for example, it is almost an immediate memory trigger of an individual who wore it.

It is also important to know that there are two sources of fragrances: (1) *natural* from plant oil extracts, and (2) *artificial* from petrochemical toxins. The artificial aroma is designed to mimic naturally-occurring scents, tricking our brains using often-toxic molecules. Although the artificial scents smell the same, the odor molecules are very different and can be quite harmful. Artificial fragrances are widely used in food, cosmetics, scented candles, and laundry products, to name a few.

Candle burning is regarded as a harmful source of airborne pollutants in indoor environments.[62] Most candles are made of paraffin wax, which creates highly toxic benzene and toluene in the air when burned. Both are known carcinogens. The toxins released from paraffin candles are the same as those found in diesel fuel fumes. Research by the Environmental Protection Agency (EPA) has shown that burning multiple candles or a candle with multiple wicks can lead to high indoor pollution levels.[63] Scented candles give off more of this soot than unscented candles. Candle burning is the new smoking. Secondhand smoke inhalation from toxic fumes from candles and incense burning indoors is worse than smoking two cigarette packs daily.

A 2001 study on candles summarizes available information on candles and incense as potential indoor air pollution sources.[64] Constant exposure to candle and incense smoke has links with several illnesses.[54] A 2014 study on emissions of lead and zinc from candles with metal core wicks estimated that burning four

Michigan-bought candles for two hours can result in airborne lead concentrations that can pose a health threat. In addition to inhalation of lead in the air, children get exposed to lead in candle fumes deposited on the floor, furniture, and walls through their hand-to-mouth activity.[65]

In a 2005 study, Netherlands' researchers measured particulate matter in churches that burn candles. Theo de Kok, PhD, of Maastricht University, found that when candles had been burning in a Dutch chapel for nine hours, particles in the air formed ten times as many free radicals as airborne particulates collected along busy roadways traveled by 45,000 vehicles daily. It also had levels of tiny, solid pollutants up to twenty times that of European limits.[56] The tiny, substantial pollutant emissions from burning candles are especially harmful because they are actual constituents of the smoke easily inhaled into the body. They readily generate free radicals, which damage cells.[66] Concentrations of the particulate matter quickly dropped after the candles were extinguished but lingered at elevated levels for twenty-four hours after simultaneous use of candles and incense.[67]

The most common ingredients used in cheap candles are fake scents. Chemicals found in petrochemical-based fragrances include phthalates, which are hormone disruptors, and benzene derivatives, aldehyde, and toluene, which are known carcinogens.

Besides the danger of toxic indoor pollution from candles, there is another reason why food-scented candle should be discouraged. Our brain and our nose cannot detect the difference between real- and fake-odor molecules. Candles are therefore a *digestive-smell miscue*. For example, when your nose smells the *phthalate-laced*, fake-vanilla-scented candle, it causes the brain to produce insulin. It also creates false anticipation of food, which can make you feel hungry when you are not.

In Alzheimer's patients, the absence of the sense of smell and taste are the first signs of the disease.[68] Alzheimer's disease affects the hippocampus and the amygdala of the brain. The amygdala plays a vital role in sending olfactory information to the hippocampus. This close connection between our olfactory nerve and the amygdala explains why Alzheimer's patients have a defective sense of smell and taste. It shuts down their appetite and sense of thirst. Typically, most Alzheimer's patients are malnourished and dehydrated because they forget to eat and drink. By contrast, an often-unintended benefit of improving one's general health is gaining a better sense of smell and taste.

Digestive Innervation

Your gut has more nerve endings than your spinal cord and your brain combined. It is the reason why any stomach imbalance will be felt intensely, often at moderate-to-severe pain levels. Most stomach pain is more intense because your gut lining is extensively guarded with pain sensors. This clever design efficiently alerts us immediately if our stomach is malfunctioning because of invaders, deficiency, or depletion.

The vagus nerve is the longest cranial nerve (CN X) connecting your brain to your gut. The vagus nerve helps manage your digestive tract's complex processes, including signaling the muscles in your stomach to contract and push food into the small intestine. A damaged vagus nerve usually cannot send signals to your stomach muscles. This may cause food to remain in your stomach longer rather than move into your small intestine to be digested. The vagus nerve and its branches can be damaged by diseases like diabetes or surgery to the stomach or small intestine.[69]

Digestion and the Enteric Nervous System

Your stomach has its own nervous system, which is called the enteric nervous system. Many neurophysiologists call it "the second brain" because the enteric nervous system can and does function autonomously. It is also essentially communicating with your central nervous system because it is influenced by your body's response, whether in the state of either parasympathetic or sympathetic nervous system.

Your gastrointestinal wall is made up of four layers of epithelial tissues. The innermost layer of epithelial tissue is formed by the mucosal layer specializing in the absorption of nutrients from chyme. The next layer is the submucosal layer that provides the blood and lymphatic vessels and nerves to support the mucosa on a surface. The next two layers of the smooth muscle are called muscularis externa are the inner circular muscular layer and the longitudinal muscular layer. And finally, the serosa layer forms the most superficial layer of your small intestines' epithelial tissues.

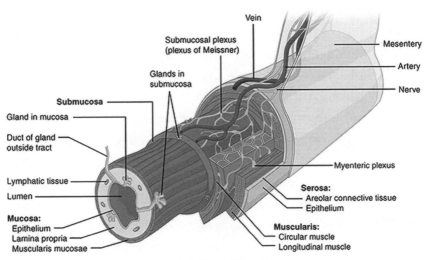

FIGURE 2.15. The Enteric Nervous System by Subhash Kulkarni [117]

The enteric nervous system's principal components are two networks or plexuses of neurons, both embedded in a digestive tract wall extending from the esophagus to the anus. It is estimated to have a hundred million neurons between the two plexuses. The first plexus is the Myenteric plexus, called Auerbach's plexus. It is a network of neurons located in the superficial areas between the longitudinal and the circular layers of muscle in the muscularis externa. Its function is to increase the gut's muscular tone, the velocity or speed, and intensity of contractions. The second plexus is the submucosal plexus, also called Meissner's plexus. As the name implies, it is buried in the submucosal or the gastrointestinal wall's innermost layer. It is involved with the local conditions and controls local secretions and blood flow to the submucosal layer. It also determines the absorption of nutrients and controls local muscle movements. The submucosal plexus is concerned with motility throughout the whole gut.

How does the enteric nervous system work in the digestive system when a person eats something? First, I will define peristalsis. Peristalsis is a series of wave-like muscle contractions that move food to different processing stations in the digestive tract.[70] The process of peristalsis begins in the esophagus when a bolus of food is swallowed. The strong wave-like motions of the smooth muscle in the esophagus carry the food to the stomach, where it is churned into a liquid mixture called chyme.[71] Next, peristalsis continues in the small intestine, where it mixes and shifts the chyme back and forth, allowing nutrients to be absorbed into the bloodstream through the small intestine walls. Peristalsis concludes in the large intestine, where water from the undigested food material is absorbed into the bloodstream. Finally, the remaining waste products are excreted from the body through the rectum and anus.

It is essential to know how the enteric nervous system controls peristalsis. It works in two different ways. First, it functions autonomously using the local reflex by coordinating the relaxation and contraction of the gastrointestinal muscles during peristalsis to efficiently absorb nutrients from the digested food or bolus while moving it toward the anus.

The second function is dependent on the sympathetic as well as the parasympathetic nervous system. Each autonomic nervous system continually communicates with the myenteric plexus and submucosal plexus, but they work opposite each other. The sympathetic nervous system stimulates the body's flight or fight response. It will be activated in case of threat, stress, and fear. In these situations, you do not need to increase gastrointestinal activity because you have to save yourself first. Therefore, the sympathetic nervous system stops or inhibits plexuses, which decreases peristalsis, decreases blood flow, reduces nutrient absorption, and decreases hydrochloric acid and local secretions in the mucosa. Meanwhile, the parasympathetic nervous system is responsible for the rest-and-digest response. When you eat a meal in a relaxed setting, your parasympathetic nervous system will be activated and stimulates both plexuses, increasing peristalsis, increasing blood flow, increasing nutrient absorption, and increasing local secretion in the mucosa.

This is the reason why when you are nervous, anxious, or afraid, your heart rate will increase, and you will feel a "knot" in your gut. For some people, they may even feel nauseated because your gut is trying to empty your stomach contents to prevent any digestion so that all the blood can be diverted to your arms and leg muscles in preparation for a sympathetic survival response–fight or flight!

DIGESTION AND TASTE

Like visual and smell appeal, the taste is fundamental in determining how well foods will be appreciated. Taste is *not* a measure of whether a food is nutritious. There are five basic tastes: sweet, sour, bitter, salty, and umami. *Umami* comes from a Japanese word, meaning *a pleasant savory taste*. According to TCM, the bitter taste has a specific function that is good for our lymphatic system, so bitter foods are crucial to our immune system.

Unfortunately, most Americans are only familiar with two kinds of tastes: sweet and salty. Processed manufactured food tricks the brain into anticipating much-needed food, causing an increase in hunger. It delivers nutrient-deficient foods, weakening an otherwise healthy diet. Sadly, the food industry is designed for profit. The more food you consume, the more profit. Processed foods are devoid of essential nutrients. I suggest that if it has a label and packaging, do not eat it!

Your taste receptors are tiny organs located mostly on the tongue, on the roof of the mouth, and at the back of the throat. The sense of smell can impact the sense of taste. For example, when one has a stuffy nose, food tends to taste bland. Interestingly, your tongue shares almost the same lining continuously down to your stomach. Your tongue is the only organ that reveals the status of your gut lining. According to TCM, your tongue's color, texture, and shape reveal whether you are healthy or not. Oriental medicine health practitioners routinely check your tongue to get a general picture of your digestion and stomach status.

FOOD TEMPERATURE AND DIGESTION

Food temperature plays a vital role in proper digestion and food experience while eating. Warm food primes the stomach for digestion. Most traditional Asian food usually starts with warm soup to promote good stomach-acid production. In his book *Practical Dietetics with Special Reference to Diet in Disease*, Dr. William Gilman Thompson, MD, PhD, stated that the ideal stomach temperature should be 98.5 °F (36.9 °C) for optimal digestion.[72] Foods taken from the refrigerator should be allowed to reach room temperature or warm-up on the stove before being eaten.

Before eating meals such as iced tea or iced-cold water, cold beverages lower the stomach's core temperature by 10°F to 20°F (−12 to −6.7°C). It, therefore, is not a good idea to start a meal with a cold beverage. A 1988 study revealed that drinking cold drinks during meals significantly slowed stomach emptying.[73] According to TCM, consuming excessively cold foods will retard or impede blood circulation in the stomach and intestines, thus slowing digestion. It is best to avoid iced cold drinks, especially around mealtime.

According to Linda Peete, RD, MS, in her book *"Just Two More Bites: Helping Picky Eaters Say Yes to Food,"* there is evidence to suggest that children who are picky eaters will sometimes improve if fed with warm, fresh foods. The author suggests that by encouraging children to play an active role in harvesting and cooking, especially when it comes to green leafy vegetables, they are more likely to eat without resistance. I experienced this when my daughters were growing up. Both of my daughters helped in the preparation of food. They both enjoyed and still enjoy fresh salads. While my daughter Ally loves broccoli, Victoria enjoys eating cherry tomatoes.

Appetite

Appetite is a desire to eat food aside from physiological needs. It is subjective mental feedback from a person's biology and awareness of food stimuli in their environment. Many factors influence appetite, including sensory responses to the sights, sounds, smells, and food tastes.

Your Satiety Center

It is essential to discuss our satiety center. The satiety center regulates the amount of food desired. Satiety is the sensation of being full. The approximate travel time of this closed-loop communication between your satiety center and when the stomach confirms the fullness sensation may take ten to fifteen minutes. The main reason you are told to eat slowly and taste every bite is so that your brain's satiety processing can catch up with your appetite.

Your hypothalamus is a part of your brain that lets you know that your stomach is full and limits further food intake. Our satiety center's pathway starts in our eyes, then our olfactory nerve stimulation through smell, then our mouth and tongue movements, then to our stomach muscles. The main trigger is when your stomach muscles are fully stretched. This stomach distension will send a message to the satiety center in the brain that it is full. It takes approximately fifteen to twenty minutes for the satiety messenger to travel from your stomach to your brain. This window of time allows us to pace our eating time gracefully and enjoy and savor every bite. When you eat too fast and too much, you do not allow enough time for the satiety communication to occur. When you are feeling bloated and overstuffed after twenty minutes of feasting on your Thanksgiving dinner, it means that your brain's satiety feedback was too late, or at worst, you overruled it. It is wise to try to eat slowly and savor your food. Eating too quickly is the most common factor in overeating.

OVEREATING

Eating the right amount of food is just as important as eating the correct type of food. When people consume more food and more calories than needed, it is called overeating. The ideal serving size per person is the size of that individual's closed fist, so it varies per person. It is just a close estimate based on your anatomical stomach size. The actual amount of food we need may not be as much as we think. Although your stomach can expand ten times when we overeat, consider that overeating greatly burdens our digestive systems, potentially leading to chronic metabolic diseases. There is overwhelming evidence from many scientific studies that suggest reduced calorie intake for most Americans promotes longevity and healthy life.[74]

Two main meals a day are adequate for most adults unless they are doing intense physical training. Studies have shown that reducing our food intake by 30 percent without compromising essential nutrients, such as vitamins, minerals, and antioxidants, will increase our lifespan by 50 percent![62] Here is a good idea for the average person: if you know you are going out for a big dinner, skip lunch and instead drink a lot of water or have a light snack. You will arrive at the dinner table with a healthy, full appetite, ready to digest the evening food in its entirety. Likewise, it is often a good idea to fast before and after feasting, such as during holiday meals. Fasting allows your body enough time and energy to digest efficiently.

We need to eat less frequently and pack our meals with adequately prepared nutrient-dense food. The frequency and timing of meals play an essential factor in our health. Eat only when you are hungry. Skip a meal if you are not hungry, but you are otherwise in good health. Food should be used solely for healthy nourishment. It should not be for emotional support. Psychological problems should be addressed instead with healthy communication, writing in a journal, or getting professional help. Taste and savor your meal by eating slowly and chewing it entirely for at least twenty to thirty times until it is almost liquid consistency before swallowing. This practice will help you pay attention to your body's signs that you are getting full. This will prevent you from overeating. Also, eating slowly allows your body to metabolize the food more efficiently, thus speeding up digestion.

CHOOSE THE RIGHT SETTING AND ATMOSPHERE FOR EATING

The right setting for meals should be a relaxed and leisurely atmosphere, preferably sitting around a dining table. As stated before, praying before meals will cue the brain to switch to the parasympathetic state, getting it ready for digestion. Dr. Emoto's studies have shown that positive intentions and prayers before meals affect the micro molecules of the food you are about to eat. Eating while working, watching TV, or driving guarantees that food will not be adequately digested. Tension and agitation disturb digestion. Therefore, upsetting subjects and distressing feelings should not be discussed at mealtimes.

In a family that dines together regularly, the children tend to be healthier and more well-adjusted. Evidence suggests that family meals influence food intake and behavior, impacting children's eating habits, diets, and health for their whole lives. Mealtimes, therefore, offer potential as settings for life-long health promotion.[75] Using real plates and silverware is ideal. By contrast, plastic utensils and plates sometimes leak toxins into your food, mostly when acidic foods are cooked in the microwave.

KNOW THE SOURCE OF YOUR FOOD

Where is your food produced? Is it from local farmers or overseas? The best way to guarantee fresh fruits and vegetables is by having homegrown or locally farmed food. Ideally, fresh produce should be harvested locally and transported within one day from the source. Overseas farming is harder to monitor in terms of whether your food is grown correctly or not. Usually, it is collected prematurely for transport to the United States. The food is not yet ripe, and, nutritionally, it is not ready to be eaten. Sometimes, it is artificially ripened with chemicals to look good in the grocery store for profit, but its nutrient content does not match that of a genuinely ripe food.

Where was your food prepared? Was it at home or in an outsourced kitchen? When you cook at home, you are more likely to choose the best ingredients. You are less likely to use artificial additives or cook junk food. Your home-cooked food quality is most often more nutritious and much better than what you would purchase pre-prepared. Also, the aroma of home cooking permeates your home and makes the experience more inviting. A home-cooked meal is guaranteed to be healthier than fast food.

According to Michael Pollan's book, entitled *Defense of Food*, *"If we outsource all our cooking to corporations, they will only buy from big companies, big farms. They are not going to buy from small farms."*[76] Big farms industrially produce meat and meal replacements. They manufacture food-like products, which are convenient and cheap. Such food-like products are big on taste, with artificial seasoning and beautiful packaging, but they are remarkably devoid of nutrients. Since they are affordable and convenient, we tend to overeat them. We become overfed and undernourished. This may be one of the major causes of the obesity epidemic and most chronic degenerative diseases.

As mentioned, in modern agricultural practice, most vegetables and fruits are picked prematurely before ripening to meet economic demand. The average transit time from field to store is between three to seven days. Most of the fresh produce may come from as far as Mexico or South America. By the time you buy your food, it is already half dead. Then, you keep it in the refrigerator for another five to seven days before you cook it. Finally, once you eat the produce, it is already approximately 75 percent dead! Studies have shown that most fruits and vegetables lose their nutrients by 50 percent when refrigerated.[77] Fresh, organic, whole food is what your body needs for optimal health. The best way is to grow your own or to purchase locally grown whole organic food from a local farmer. Not only is it good for your health, but it helps the local economy.

EAT WHAT IS IN SEASON

All living organisms, from plants to animals, are in sync with Mother Nature's rhythm. Ancient civilizations knew and lived by the biorhythm of the earth and seasonal changes. The foods that were eaten reflected what was in season. Plants and animals are in synchrony with the seasons. Vegetables and fruits have their nutritional peak according to their seasonal timing. The modern monoculture and global farming have deprived most American families of determining which seasons are for which vegetables and fruits.

When do you eat certain vegetables and fruits? If you do not already, consider eating what is in season. Your body has a physiological biorhythm. Our body's physiological needs change with the season. Unfortunately, most Americans only eat nine favorite fruits and vegetables over and over. All sorts of different vegetables from all over the world are conveniently available in grocery stores all year round, regardless of the season. Most of my patients will eat the same vegetables for years, without variety. Eating like this is not suitable for you. It eventually causes food intolerance and leads to food allergies or even leaky gut problems.

A classic example happened when kale was hailed as a superfood a few years back. I had a patient who drank only kale smoothies all year round for five years or more. When she came to the clinic for gut problems, I tested her blood for food allergies and intolerances. The test showed that all the fruits and vegetables she repeatedly ate for years had caused inflammation in her body, even the good, "almighty" kale! We need to stay in sync with the seasons, especially when it comes to vegetable and fruit consumption. To prevent depletion and deficiency of nutrients, we need a balanced diet and a variety of foods that follow the three-month seasonal cycle.

When I was a kid, growing up in a tropical country, my local environment gave me a frequent hint about what was in season, both in vegetables and fruits. I always looked forward to the abundant fruit in the summer season, which would appear in the public market and on the streets. You could enjoy the delicious taste of seasonal fruits like mangoes, jackfruits, durians, lansones, and other vegetables. There is also seasonal ocean meat. I remember that we could only eat what was in season in the ocean, like the famous Oroquieta squid. Its peak harvest happens only during the summer.

FOOD LABEL

The *USDA Organic* label generally means that a product has relatively minimal synthetic pesticides and fertilizers and that animals are bred according to specific government guidelines. Fraud in organic labeling has plagued the system. My rule of thumb on original labels: if the food is farmed organically in

America, you can count on it being roughly 90 percent organically farmed. For organic produce farmed outside the United States, it may vary significantly despite having the organic label. Use your judgment, and buyer beware!

There is a new and better farming practice called biodynamic farming. Biodynamic plants are grown in the ground in living soil, which provides a higher level of nutrition not possible with chemical fertilizers or hydroponic growing. Biodynamic farms aspire to generate their fertility through composting, integrating animals, covering crops, and rotating crops.[78] Look for biodynamic labels in your grocery stores or local farmer's market.

A survey on American children at school was done on their basic knowledge of vegetables and fruits.[79] The survey found that the children had a hard time with five key concepts: (1) they could not identify fruits and vegetables; (2) they did not know when to plant and harvest; (3) they did not know when fruits and vegetables reached their fullest nutritional value; (4) they also had a hard time identifying when they are ripe to eat; and (5) they could not match the plant with its corresponding fruit or vegetable. Sadly, these schoolchildren were being served only three popular vegetables from their state-prepared American school meals. They are tomatoes in pizza, lettuce in burgers, and potatoes in French fries. No wonder our children are suffering from degenerative diseases and attention deficits. It is appalling.

There is hope. A 2010 study in Baton Rouge, Louisiana, showed that by repeatedly tasting vegetables between eight to nine times, children reported liking, or like a lot, previously disliked vegetables or less-liked vegetables that were served in a cafeteria-based setting.[80] This study proved that we need to expose our kids more consistently and repeatedly to a variety of vegetables, regardless of their initial feedback. Home economics, gardening, and healthy food preparation should return to the curriculum. Children should be taught the basic hands-on knowledge of vegetables and fruits, from planting seeds to tasting fresh foods while they harvest. This is critical for the health and future of our children.

EAT EARLY, NOT LATE

When is the best time of day to eat? Our circadian rhythms, metabolism, and nutrition are intimately linked.[81] Eating in sync with cycles of the sun is critical to proper digestion. The timing of our meals is vital. Your most substantial meal should be eaten preferably in the morning or the afternoon, not late at night.

It is best to eat during daylight hours and, at the latest, two hours after sundown. This is true, especially for women, whose biorhythms are designed to be more in sync with the sun. Many of the female hormones follow their circadian rhythm.

If that is not possible, be sure to have dinner in the early part of the evening and not eat again before bedtime. If you must eat in the latter part of the evening, go for a walk or gently move your body in some other way after the meal. This will help stimulate the digestive process, especially if you have overeaten.

Eating a large meal late at night makes it impossible to sleep properly. It affects the circadian regulation of plasma glucose and triglyceride concentration in your liver.[82] It could lead to indigestion and the unhealthy fermentation of food in your gut, leaving you gassy or with heartburn. A large meal before bed will keep your digestive system working all night. It also prevents the liver from expelling the toxins in the blood, resulting in feeling tired and hungover when you wake up the next day.

FOOD PREPARATION AND DIGESTION

How fresh should your food be? Raw and recently harvested food is always healthy. Fresh food properly cooked and prepared is ideal. Refrigeration does not prevent the loss of essential food nutrients. Fresh is not frozen. Once harvested, fruits and vegetables will rapidly deteriorate and oxidize, resulting in a decline in their nutritional value stored for more than a few days. According to Barbara P. Klein, PhD, a Food Science and Human Nutrition professor at the University of Illinois at Urbana-Champaign, most farmers' produce has usually already spent days in transport and on display shelves. Once they hit the refrigerator, some fruits and vegetables can lose as much as 50 percent of their vitamin C and other nutrients in the following week, depending on the temperature.[83]

When I was growing up, we did not have electricity. We did not own a refrigerator. We went to the local market to buy our food daily. Fruits and vegetables were seasonal from local farms or neighbors' backyards. We always had fresh vegetables and fruits and fresh wild-caught fish, depending on what was in season. Ironically, it was how poor people lived. I did not realize how lucky I was.

Ideally, healthy, green, leafy vegetables should be eaten raw to benefit from the live enzymes they contain. Most animal-based protein must be adequately cooked unless you like your steak raw like steak tar-tar. If you must cook, the preferred methods are steaming, poaching, baking, and stir-frying. *Avoid overcooking*: broiling, cooking over charcoal, deep-frying, and microwaving. I will elaborate more on food preparation in Chapter 9 in Book Three, *Understanding How Epigenetics Heals You,* but in short, overcooking can deteriorate the food nutrients. The longer you cook it, the higher the nutrient losses. For example, nutrients like vitamins B and C are lost when foods are boiled or soaked in water, and the water is thrown away. Most vegetables, such as spinach, carrots, and broccoli, are healthier eaten raw or slightly cooked.

The next chapter is about your microbiome. Your guest microbes are great helpers to your body.

 Your gut's digestion is the engine for your health.

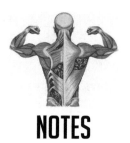

NOTES

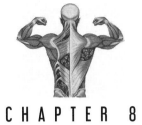

CHAPTER 8
YOUR MICROBIOTA

"When diet is wrong, medicine is of no use. When diet is correct, medicine is of no need."
—Hippocrates

W hen we hear the words "microbes," "bacteria," or "viruses," we tend to think of something terrible, but not all microorganisms are harmful. Your body is home to trillions of bacteria and other microbes, collectively known as your "microbiome." The word "microbiome" refers to the village or community of microorganisms and their genes which reside in your body. The microbiota is the microbes themselves. The microbiota is the individual citizens of the village.

In 2007, the National Institutes of Health (NIH) launched the Human Microbiome Project (HMP) as a conceptual extension of the Human Genome Project to study the human body as a *supraorganism* composed of both nonhuman and human cells. A 2012 study by the HMP Consortium found that there might be more than 8 million unique microbial genes inside the human body.[84] This means that as a *supraorganism* human, you have more nonhuman microbes than human cells. The number of genes in all the microbes in one person's microbiota is 200 times the number of genes in the human genome.[85] The genome's primary function is to store, propagate, and express the genetic information that gives rise to a cell's blueprint for its architectural and functional machinery.

MICROBIOTA

You are covered in microorganisms! Your body has more microbes than human cells. You can find trillions of them in many sites of your body, including your skin (especially the moist areas, such as the groin and between the toes), your respiratory tract (particularly the nose), your urinary tract, your genitals (lining of the vagina), your gut and your digestive tract (primarily the mouth and the colon).[86] On the other hand, there are microbe-free or sterile areas, such as the brain, the circulatory system, and the lungs.

Microbes started to populate your body during birth or shortly after that.[87] Your microbiota comes from your mother during vaginal delivery.[88] As you arrive into the world, you are immunized with your mother's bacteria to boost your immune system. The next best route to enhance your microbiota is breastfeeding. Human breast milk is the best way to boost an infant's immune systems to the fullest. Mature human milk contains 3–5 percent fat, 0.8–0.9 percent protein, 6.9–7.2 percent carbohydrate calculated as lactose, and 0.2 percent mineral constituents expressed as ash.[89] The rest is approximately 85 percent water. If possible, the longer you breastfeed, the better fortification it is for your infant's immune system. Ideally, it is best to breastfeed for a year or up until your baby will be able to eat balanced and nutritious solid food.

Your microbiotas are like house guests in your body. They are highly trained microorganisms like bacteria, viruses, and fungi that live on and inside you. They have a harmless symbiotic or mutualistic relationship with your cells. Your body provides many unique environments for different bacterial communities. In return for hosting and feeding them in your body, they work many jobs to maintain your optimal health. This symbiotic relationship benefits both the host (your body) and the microbes (your house guests). They are your body's super helpers!

Most of the beneficial microbes in the microbiome do not cause disease. However, the host-microbe relationship can be healthy, neutral, or harmful. It becomes destructive only when the host-microbe relationship becomes parasitic (in which case the microbe takes advantage of the host) or pathogenic (the microbe causes damage to the host). In pathogenic relationships, the opportunistic germs that cause disease take advantage of the beneficial bacteria when the immune system is weakened within the host's natural flora. In both cases, the cost to the host's health can vary from very mild to catastrophic. It is to your advantage to maintain a healthy, balanced relationship with the vibrant ecosystem of your microbiota.

Although the essential functions of individual microbes within our bodies are not fully understood, we are heavily dependent on microbes to perform many critical tasks that our cells cannot perform. Your microbes play all the typical *housekeeping* properties for maintaining cell function. Microbes digest food to generate nutrients for host cells, synthesize vitamins, metabolize drugs, detoxify carcinogens, stimulate the renewal of cells in the gut lining, and activate and support the immune system.[90]

It is essential to establish and define what makes a healthy microbiome. Your microbial health has significant implications for your health. Two crucial factors constitute a healthy microbiome: microbial diversity and the health status of the microbiome. Microbial diversity is dependent on the microbial population, either high or low, and dependent on the body-site location. However, it is even more relevant to check the microbes' health and determine whether their function is disrupted or weakened in strength. This is more predictive of disease or good health than microbial diversity because microbial diversity can fluctuate, depending on the individual's diet or environment. Still, they are not necessarily symptomatic right away.[91]

Skin Microbiota

The skin is the second most common body site for microbes, next to the gut. Skin microbiotas are microorganisms that colonize your skin. A thin microlayer of organisms protects your skin. Your skin surface is relatively dry and slightly acidic. This slightly acidic environment prevents the growth of many microorganisms, but a few have adapted to live on your skin. Your dead skin cells are the primary source of nutrition for your microbiota.[92] Your skin microbiota can prevent the colonization of other pathogenic microbes by using up the nutritional sources that those harmful microbes require to survive and producing toxic substances that stop the pathogens from adhering to skin cells.[93]

Speaking of skin microbiota, the Human Microbiome Project (HMP) Consortium investigators have found that the microbes are not the same across the body and are different from person to person. Researchers found that the higher likelihood of similarity between microbial communities was body-site-specific rather than body specific. For example, between two subjects, microbes on the first subject's skin were the most similar to the bacteria on the second subject's skin, regardless of their gender. They also found a site-specific similarity between men and women. Interestingly, even twins can have different microbiomes composition. Despite twins potentially having shared the same human genetics, individually, they have diverse microbiomes' genetic makeup.

More than ever, in this pandemic climate, it is essential to be careful in applying any products on your skin that contain antimicrobial compounds, like 99 percent alcohol or triclosan in hand-sanitizer gels or soaps. They can effectively wipe out your skin microbiota balance. They can leave your skin dry and leave skin pores unprotected, becoming susceptible to pathogenic invasion. Interestingly, the link between handwashing and the spread of disease was established two centuries ago. It is the most effective medical practice of infection control, also known as "hand hygiene." It is hand washing with soap and water. It is best to use regular soap for handwashing. Regular soaps used daily are mild enough not to hurt your skin microbiota but strong enough to kill pathogens.

Gut Microbiota

In this section, I will use the term "gut bacteria" to refer to all microorganisms or bacteria that live in the entire region of your digestive tract. Your gut microbiota is made up of trillions of bacteria, fungi, and other microbes that reside in your digestive tract. Your gut lining hosts five pounds of them! Surprisingly, these microorganisms can live in a highly acidic (pH 1 to 2) environment of your gut. The bacteria safely inhabit your gut by burrowing into the stomach's mucosal lining to a depth where the pH is mostly neutral. Your gut bacteria perform essential digestive functions 24/7.

Your gut-bacteria colony helps in digestion by breaking down food that the body cannot otherwise digest. Your gut bacteria can also help make essential nutrients for your body if your gut provides a home and nutrition for the colonizing microbe. The microbe occupies space that serves as a significant intestinal barrier, preventing a potential parasite or pathogen that might have otherwise colonized your gut. Your gut controls and deals with every aspect of your health. How you digest your food and even your food sensitivities are linked with your mood, behavior, energy, weight, food cravings, hormone balance, immunity, and overall wellness.[94]

Although we are born without bacteria in the colon, it is quickly acquired through breastfeeding or bottle feeding. The number of bacteria in the colon far outnumber the number in the small intestine. Bacteria can be found in any of these areas of the large intestine. In your colon, bacteria account for about 35 to 50 percent of your colon contents, amounting to approximately two pounds of total body weight in an adult,[95] the colon is the place where the end stages of food digestion occur. For it is here that a massive amount of your gut bacteria is being stored and, most importantly, where the bulk of the microbial work happens. As an aid in digestion, bacteria in the colon also help the body absorb nutrients that would have been otherwise lost. Biotin and vitamin K are absorbed primarily, thanks to the assistance of bacteria in the colon.[96]

The outdated medical dogma that your appendix is *"useless"* needs to be updated. It has only been recently recognized that your appendix is a vital organ for developing and preserving the intestinal immune system. It contributes to the balancing of your intestinal pro- and anti-inflammatory activity for maintaining homeostasis in your gut. Since your gut microbiome composition can vary over the short-term and long-term, your appendix is instrumental in maintaining the intestinal microbiome.[97] A recent study has highlighted that your appendix may have a significant association with chronic diseases, particularly in developing large-bowel cancer following the appendix's surgical removal.[98] Moreover, a study was done on appendectomy's relationship to mood disorders; it postulated that an appendectomy might lead to psychological disturbances.[99]

The state of your gut microbiota can change the expression of your genes' DNA. Many factors affect your microbiota, including your environment, medications such as antibiotics, or whether or not you were delivered by C-section. The state of your microbiota is strongly linked to your epigenetic consequences. You can manipulate the balance of your microbes by paying attention to what you eat. Gut health can be nurtured through the daily consumption of raw probiotics and prebiotic fibers, also known as vegetable fibers. Dietary fiber from fruits and vegetables, nuts, legumes, and whole grains is the best fuel for gut bacteria. It is especially beneficial to select organic or biodynamically farmed foods to enhance good bacteria's growth and minimize low-dose exposure to pesticides and antibiotics.

A recent study of clinically treated patients with antibiotics for appendicitis increased the risk of large-bowel cancer significantly.[100] It is critical to point out that even a single dose of antibiotics will decimate your entire gut bacterial balance like a nuclear bomb. Every single round of antibiotics may take at least a year or two to be reinoculated again with a proper gut balance between good and bad bacteria. According to a 2012 study, supplemental probiotics help treat and prevent antibiotic-associated symptoms.[101] It is, therefore, essential to supplement with probiotics after antibiotic therapy aggressively.

PROBIOTICS

Probiotics are substances infused with live microorganisms that help support the growth of the right bacterial balance in your gut. They contain beneficial live bacteria, which are naturally created by the process of fermentation. Probiotics are the most important supplement you need to acquire either from food or OTC supplements for maintaining optimal health.[102] They help your gut replenish good bacteria and control harmful bacteria.

I often see people follow only part of the protocol in healing their gut by removing certain damaging irritants. But the part they often leave out is reinoculating their stomachs with beneficial bacteria that will keep harmful bacteria at bay. So, load up on probiotic-rich foods. If you must take oral supplements rather than obtain it through food, take at least 50 billion units of probiotics daily from a high-quality brand on an empty stomach at night or first thing in the morning.[103] However, with live beneficial bacteria, the best probiotics can be sourced from raw food through fermentation.

PREBIOTICS

Prebiotics are a form of dietary fiber that acts as a fertilizer for the good bacteria in your gut. They feed the good bacteria colonies in your stomach. They help increase the number of desirable bacteria in your gut, associated with better health and reduced disease risk. Prebiotic fiber goes through the small intestine undigested. Fermentation happens in the large colon.

Prebiotic fiber is the nondigestible part of foods like bananas, onions and garlic, Jerusalem artichokes, apples, chicory root, and beans. Even tea, coffee, red wine, and dark chocolate are correlative with increased bacterial diversity. In a 2016 study, led by geneticist Cisco Warming, PhD, professor of Human Genetics, researchers analyzed 1,135 stool samples. They identified some beneficial foods for gut-microbiota diversity. In addition to fruits and vegetables, they found that nuts, coffee, tea, and red wine favored the variety of bacteria.[104] These foods contain polyphenols, which are naturally occurring antioxidant compounds that support your gut flora. On the other hand, diets with foods high on sugar content and especially in the form of sugar-sweetened drinks, such as sodas, were correlated with decreased microbial diversity.

Fresh organic vegetables and fruits are the best sources of prebiotic fiber. They should be free from pesticides and antibiotic loads, which may harm your gut's natural flora. Minimally processed fresh food generally contains more fibers and provides better fuel. Vegetables lightly steamed, sautéed, or raw are typically more beneficial than fried.

FERMENTATION

Long before electricity and refrigeration were invented, fermentation was widely practiced in many ancient cultures for hundreds of years. It is an ancient technique in preserving food. Fermentation is a process that involves the breakdown of carbohydrates by bacteria and yeast into alcohol and acids. The alcohol and acids act as natural preservatives. They also give the fermented food its distinctive tart flavor. Fermented food is teaming with healthful probiotic bacteria like *lactobacilli*, *bifidobacteria*, and many more. Fermentation is used to make foods like wine, kombucha, kimchi, tempeh, cheese, and sauerkraut.

A 2018 study showed strong evidence for the positive impact of fermented foods and beverages, such as yogurt, pickles, bread, kefir, beers, wines, and mead. They are produced or preserved by the action of microorganisms using ancient sea salt or yeast organisms. Fermented foods play a vital role in gut-microbiota balance and brain function.[105] Consistent consumption of vibrant probiotics, especially those contained in fermented foods, is found to have significant improvement in your intestine's ability to protect itself from harm and to soak up nutrients.[106]

Traditionally, there were two reasons for fermentation: survival and nutritional health. The first reason was for survival or economic purposes. During the summer or early fall, fruits and vegetables were plentiful from the farm and garden. Fermentation was done to extend the availability of these foods for the upcoming leaner winter months.

The second reason was for nutritional health. As mentioned, fermentation promotes the growth of beneficial bacteria known as *probiotics*. It improves your digestive and heart health, in addition to strengthening your immune system. Therefore, eating fermented foods daily will help you achieve optimal health.[82] Fermentation fortifies the gut against diseases. Many foods are much more nutritious when fermented than in their unfermented form. Fermented foods have active enzymes from the ingredient materials interacting with the metabolic activities of the fermenting organisms.[107] It is the most ancient way of infusing your foods with billions of beneficial microorganisms. Your microbial helpers "*hitchhike*" on fermented food to enter your gut. I suspect our ancestors knew this all along.

When milk lactose is fermented, the lactose, which is the natural sugar molecule in milk, is broken down into simple sugars: glucose and galactose. Since fermented milk products, like cheese, kefir, and yogurt, are thus rendered lactose free, even genetically lactose-intolerant people can eat them without experiencing uncomfortable symptoms. Besides, these products are so much healthier for you. A 2018 study done in Spain found that the consumption of totally fermented dairy products was associated with a better-quality diet, evidenced by a significant reduction of the participants' cardio-metabolic profile (or heart and gut health).[108]

Yogurt is a prevalent fermented food that can introduce helpful bacteria into your gut. However, make sure it has low sugar content, less than five grams. Otherwise, it may contain too much sugar and not enough bacteria.

Dried legumes, beans, grains, and seeds all contain the protective antinutrient enzymes called *phytates* and *lectins*. As is (that is, without soaking or fermenting them), they are so difficult to digest that, for some people, they destroy their gut lining. As discussed previously, phytates and lectins are two of the leading causes of the leaky gut syndrome and possibly autoimmune diseases. This protective design is mother nature's way of preserving their future generation. It is a form of biochemical protection, and it is why these food items do not grow or root when stored in your pantry. Fermentation helps break down antinutrients and unleash their beneficial nutrients.

In many Asian cuisines, you find tempeh, fermented bean natto, fermented soybeans, as well as soy sauce, and kimchi. Europeans consume a lot of sauerkraut and wine. Wine comes from fermented grapes that contain a beneficial polyphenol called *resveratrol*. *Resveratrol* in wine has positive effects, such as improved antioxidant capacity and modulating inflammation of the brain.[109] Additional sources of fermented foods include beer, which is fermented barley, and vodka, which is fermented cereal grains or potatoes.

For centuries, fermentation has been practiced. Recent controlled scientific investigations support these traditional practices. They confirm that probiotics are a valuable part of our healthy diet.[110] Fermented foods are beneficial to our heart health by lowering our blood pressure, improving heart-blood circulation, and reducing inflammation around the arteries and veins.[96]

Many scientific studies have proven for years that the gut-brain connection is vital to our survival. Gut-brain connection begins with fermenting our food.[111] Why? Because the human body consists of approximately 10 percent of human cells and 90 percent of bacteria, or non-human cells. Fermentation has so many compelling health benefits because it gives us life-boosting probiotics. I recommend reading Dr. Perlmutter's books: *Grain Brain and Brain Maker*, for starters. It elaborates on how different probiotics enhance all the physiological processes in the human body.

Now I would like to mention a few of the beneficial bacteria naturally found in probiotic foods. Such foods include Italian and Swiss cheeses (Parmesan, cheddar, and Gruyère), milk, kefir, and buttermilk. Fermented foods (kombucha, kimchi, pickles, olives, and sauerkraut), with *Lactobacillus Helveticas* and *Bifidobacterium longum,* help our brain in reducing anxiety and depression.[112] According to Dr. Perlmutter, these probiotics actively protect our brain from most neurodegenerative diseases, such as Alzheimer's disease, dementia, and Parkinson's disease.[113] It is interesting to note that the early symptoms of Parkinson's disease are gut issues, such as diarrhea, bloating, and poor digestion. *Lactobacillus rhamnosus* and *Lactobacillus gasseri,* according to some researchers, are strains of probiotics that help with weight loss and in reducing belly fat.[114]

Modern lifestyles have taken us away from practicing fermentation. If you are too busy to ferment on your own, oral supplementation may be your best bet. There are so many kinds of probiotic supplements on the market that choosing one can be confusing. Make sure you do your due-diligence research before choosing. There are so many reliable sources to draw from in this regard, such as recommendations from the giants of preventive medicine like Dr. Mercola, DO, and Dr. Perlmutter, MD.

GUT-BRAIN SCIENCE: PSYCHONEUROIMMUNOLOGY

I am so excited to elaborate on a relatively new field of study in medicine. Psychoneuroimmunology (PNI) studies the interaction between the nervous system's psychological processes and the immune systems. It is also referred to as psychoendoneuroimmunology (PENI) or psychoneuroendocrinoimmunology (PNEI).

Psychoneuroimmunology studies the brain, heart, and gut connection. It is the close connection between the foods you eat, your emotions, your mind, and your immune system. There are a direct correlation and causation between your diet, your immune system, and the amount of perceived stress in your life. The quality of your stress-coping mechanism determines your overall health.

Your stress response is massively dependent on how healthy your gut microbiota is from your diet. I recently learned a helpful formula for understanding life:

EVENTS + RESPONSE = OUTCOME [E+R=O]

Simply put, your life's EVENTS, in addition to your RESPONSE to your circumstances, predict what kind of OUTCOME or experience you are going to live. Your response to life's events is the single determining factor on how happy and fulfilled you are.

Essentially, you have three brains in your body: head brain, heart brain, and gut-brain (see Figure 2.16). These three brains cross-communicate with each other every nanosecond 24/7. Each organ has complex neural networks and can store and process information. Each brain has the capacity for neuroplasticity. The brain in your head is made up of 100 billion neurons. In 1991, neurocardiologist Dr. J. Andrew Armour, MD, discovered that the heart has its "little brain" or "intrinsic cardiac nervous system." This "heart brain" comprises approximately 40,000 neurons that are similar neurons in the brain, meaning that the heart has its nervous system.[115] Your heart also acts as a heart brain, which can sense, feel, learn, and remember. The heart sends more information to the brain than the brain sends to the heart.

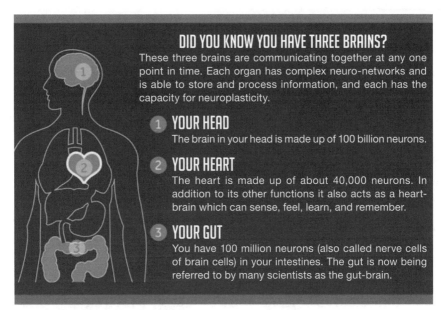

DID YOU KNOW YOU HAVE THREE BRAINS?

These three brains are communicating together at any one point in time. Each organ has complex neuro-networks and is able to store and process information, and each has the capacity for neuroplasticity.

① YOUR HEAD

The brain in your head is made up of 100 billion neurons.

② YOUR HEART

The heart is made up of about 40,000 neurons. In addition to its other functions it also acts as a heart-brain which can sense, feel, learn, and remember.

③ YOUR GUT

You have 100 million neurons (also called nerve cells of brain cells) in your intestines. The gut is now being referred to by many scientists as the gut-brain.

FIGURE 2.16. THE THREE BRAINS IN YOUR BODY

And finally, the brain in your gut is lined with more than 100 million nerve cells—it's practically a brain unto itself. The enteric nervous system is often referred to as our body's third brain. There are hundreds of millions of neurons connecting the brain to the enteric nervous system, which is part of the nervous system tasked with controlling the gastrointestinal system. The gut is now being referred to by many scientists as the gut-brain.

According to gut-brain science, it is proven that your gut microbiota sends signals to your brain as to what kind of food to crave and eat. Your gut actually talks to your brain, releasing hormones into the bloodstream that, over the course of about 10 minutes, tells you how hungry it is or that you should not have eaten an entire pizza. Indeed, your microbiota's healthy food cravings signify a healthy immune system. Your neurotransmitters— serotonin, dopamine, and endorphins—are your "happy" and "resilient" neurotransmitters that positively help your brain process life's events. Your gut manufactures 90 percent of blood serotonin and endorphins, as well as about 50 percent of the body's dopamine.[116]

Once your gut is healthy, it will produce an unlimited supply of necessary neurotransmitters for a healthy body and balanced emotions. You will be more resilient with better neurotransmitters; a healthy outcome equals a healthy and happy life!

GUT AS THE NEUROTRANSMITTER FACTORY

Neurologist Dr. Perlmutter, MD, promotes the idea that your brain maker is your gut. Nurturing gut health feeds the brain and the entire body. Now there is proper and extensive research on the brain-and-gut connection. As mentioned previously, your stomach manufactures most of what your brain needs, such as serotonin, dopamine, and all other neurotransmitters. Neurotransmitters are simply brain messengers produced in your gut. Your brain is the mainly consumer of all the crucial neurotransmitters. It is not the producer. When your gut is provided with the right raw materials,

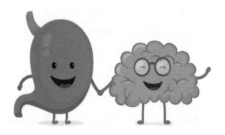

FIGURE 2.17. THE GUT-BRAIN SCIENCE

your stomach makes what the brain needs. Your stomach makes neurotransmitters and feeds good bacteria from the healthy vegetables and organic, pasture-raised meats you consume.

It is important to note that anyone who begins to feel any anxiety or depression should primarily address what they are putting in their gut. Eating junk foods will cause a depletion of nutrients and will not nourish or sustain brain health. People simply do not realize that whatever is put on your plate will essentially become parts of the brain and body. Healthy food creates a functioning brain, while junk food creates a junk brain. Studies have shown that gut-bacterial balance changes may cause diabetes, multiple sclerosis, Parkinson's, anxiety, ADHD, ADD, and even depression.[101,100] An absence or decrease of good bacteria in the gut increases inflammation and oxidative stress, potentially causing many chronic degenerative diseases.

 Your microbiomes are your body's guest workers for optimal health.

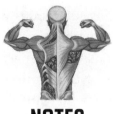

NOTES

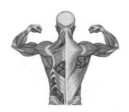

BOOK 2 SUMMARY HIGHLIGHTS

Chapter 5: Epigenetics changes happen in your nucleus and your mitochondria. Your cell membrane controls what comes in and out of your cells.

Chapter 6: Your self-healing system: autonomic nervous system, meridians, lymphatic system, and digestive system

Chapter 7: Your gut's digestion is the engine for your health.

Chapter 8: Your microbiomes are your body's guest workers for optimal health.

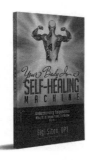 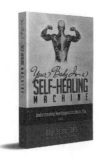

Now that you have finished Book One, *"Understanding Epigenetics – Why It Is Important to Know,"* had chapters 1 to 4, and Book Two, *"Understanding the Anatomy of Epigenetics,"* had chapters 5 to 8. You have gained a solid epigenetic groundwork, a good foundation for

the last book of the Epigenetic trilogy. I am sure you are excited about how to incorporate all the epigenetic knowledge into your daily life. Coming up, Book Three, *"Understanding How Epigenetics Heals You,"* has chapters 9 to 15. You will learn more practical epigenetic solutions. The trilogy's final book will explain how to use epigenetics for you and your family to achieve optimal health.

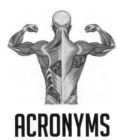

ACRONYMS

ACERO	Aberdeen Centre for Energy Regulation and Obesity
ADD	Attention Deficit Disorder
ADHD	Attention Deficit Hyperactivity Disorder
AGD	Anogenital Distance
AFO	Animal Feeding Operations
ALA	Alpha Linolenic Acid
AM	Amplitude Modulation
ANS	Autonomic Nervous System
ARA	Adenine Arabinoside
ATP	Adenosine Triphosphate
BAP	British Association of Psychopharmacology
BALT	Bronchial-associated Lymphoid Tissue
BBM	Buteyko Breathing Medicine
BBT	Buteyko Breathing Technique
BHA	Butylated Hydroxyanisole
BHT	Butylated Hydroxytoluene
BPA	Bisphenol A
CAFOS	Confined Animal Feeding Operations
CCK	Cholecystokinin
CD	Celiac Disease
CDC	Centers for Disease Control and Prevention

CKD	Cyclic Ketogenic Diet
CLA	Conjugated Linoleic Acid
COPD	Chronic Obstructive Pulmonary Disease
CSF	Cerebrospinal Fluid
CST	Craniosacral Therapy
CT	Computer Tomography
DGLA	Dihomogamma-linolenic Acid
DNA	Deoxyribonucleic Acid
DH	Dermatitis Herpetiformis
DHA	Docosahexaenoic Acid
DSM	Diagnostic and Statistical Manual of Mental Disorders
ECG	Electrocardiogram
ECT	Electroconvulsive Therapy
ED	Erectile Dysfunction
EGF	Epidermal Growth Factor
EMG	Electromyograph
EMF	Electromagnetic Field
EPA	Environmental Protection Agency
EPA	Eicosapentaenoic Acid
EWG	Environmental Working Group
FAO	Food and Agriculture Organization of the United Nations
FDA	Food and Drug Administration
FM	Frequency Modulation
FPG	Fasting Plasma Glucose
GABA	Gamma-aminobutyric Acid
GALT	Gut-associated Lymphoid Tissue
GERD	Gastroesophageal Reflux Disease
GLA	Gamma Linolenic Acid

GMO	Genetically Modified Organism
HDL	High Density Lipoproteins
HMP	Human Microbiome Project
HPKD	High Protein Ketogenic Diet
IBS	Irritable Bowel Syndrome
IF	Intermittent Fasting
IGF	Insulin-like Growth Factor
IM	Innovative Medicine
LDL	Low Density Lipoproteins
MCT	Medium Chain Triglyceride
MnSOD	Manganese-dependent Superoxide Dismutase
MRSA	Methicillin-resistant Staphylococcus Aureus
MS	Multiple Sclerosis
mV	milliVolts
NASA	National Aeronautics and Space Administration
NAFLD	Nonalcoholic Fatty Liver Disease
NCGS	Nonceliac Gluten Sensitivity
NIH	National Institutes of Health
NLFES	Nonionizing Low Frequency Electromagnetic Waves
NM	Neural Manipulation
NSAIDs	Nonsteroidal Anti-inflammatory Drugs
OTC	Over The Counter
PCOS	Polycystic Ovary Syndrome
PDE	Phosphodiesterase
PEFR	Peak Respiratory Flow Rate
PENI	Psychoendocrinoimmunology
PFOA	Perflourooctanoic Acid
PNEI	Psychoneuroendocrinoimmunology
PNI	Psychoneuroimmunology
PPI	Proton Pump Inhibitors

PT	Physical Therapy
PTH	Parathyroid Hormone
PTSD	Post-Traumatic Stress Disorder
RBC	Red Blood Cell
rBGH	Recombinant Bovine Growth Hormone
REM	Rapid Eye Movement
RNA	Ribonucleic Acid
ROM	Range of Motion
ROS	Reactive Oxygen Species
SAD	Seasonal Affective Disorder
SAM	Sulfur-adenosylmethionine dismutase
SCN	Suprachiasmatic Nucleus
SIAM	Italian Society of Andrology and Sexual Medicine
SKD	Standard Ketogenic Diet
SLES	Sodium Laureth Sulfate
SLS	Sodium Lauryl Sulfate
TBHQ	Tertiary Butylhydroquinone
TCM	Traditional Chinese Medicine
TEA	Triethanomaline
TKD	Targeted Ketogenic Diet
UHT	Ultra-heat Treated
USDA	United States Department of Agriculture
UTHSC	University of Tennessee Health Science Center
VM	Visceral Manipulation
VRA	Vancomycin-resistant Enterococcus
WBC	White Blood Cell
WHO	World Health Organization
XEs	Xenoestrogens

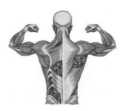

REFERENCES

1   Dunne, J.L., Triplett, E.W., Gevers, D., Xavier, R., Insel, R., Danska, J., Atkinson, M.A.: The Intestinal Microbiome in Type 1 Diabetes. Clinical and Experimental Immunology 177(1):30-7, 2014.

2   https://www.genome.gov/genetics-glossary/histone, extracted October 31, 2020

3   Bruce Lipton, PhD, Insight into Cellular Consciousness, Thu, June 7, 2012, Reprinted from Bridges, 2001 Vol 12(1):5 ISSEEM

4   Steven Goodman, PhD, Goodman's Medical Cell Biology, Fourth Edition, Academic Press, Elsevier, June 2020

5   https://opentextbc.ca/anatomyandphysiology/chapter/the-cell-membrane

6   Know Your Fats Book, by Mary G. Enig, PhD

7   www.westonaprice.org – Articles: "The Skinny on Fat" and "Fats and Oils FAQ's," "The Great Con-ola," by Mary G. Enig, PhD and Sally Fallon; Nutritional Therapy Association, Inc., "Fatty Acids Module – NTT Curriculum."

8   https://www.mayoclinic.org/diseases-conditions/dehydration/symptoms-causes/syc-20354086

9   Kirsch, Daniel, PhD, chapter author on Electromedicine: The Other Side of Physiology, and A Practical Protocol for Electromedical Treatment of Pain in the American Academy of Pain Management's textbook, Pain Management: A Practical Guide for Clinicians (CRC Press, Boca Raton, Florida, 2002)

10 Voet, D., et al (2006). Fundamentals of Biochemistry, 2nd Edition, John Wiley and Sons, Inc.

11 G. Schatz. The Magic Garden. Annu. Rev. Biochem. 2007. 76:673-78, http://www.life.sci.qut.edu.au/epping/LQB381ScROLL/Fronteirs_reviews/mitochondria.pdf

12 Davies, KJ. Oxidative stress: the paradox of aerobic life Biochem Soc Symp. 1995;61:1-31. http://www.ncbi.nlm.nih.gov/pubmed/8660387

13 "The Care and Feeding of Your Mitochondria", by Pamela Weintraub, March 27, 2019 https://experiencelife.com/article/the-care-and-feeding-of-your-mitochondria

14 Terry Wahls M.D., The Wahls Protocol: A Radical New Way to Treat All Chronic, Eve Adamson - 2014

15 Sivitz WI, Yorek MA. Mitochondrial dysfunction in diabetes: from molecular mechanisms to functional significance and therapeutic opportunities. Antioxid Redox Signal. 2010;12(4):537-577. doi:10.1089/ars.2009.2531

16 The Care and Feeding of Your Mitochondria," by Pamela Weintraub, March 27, 2019 https://experiencelife.com/article/the-care-and-feeding-of-your-mitochondria

17 The Effects of Electromagnetic Fields on Mitochondria: An Ultrastructural and Biochemical Study Najam Siddiqi, Naseer Salem Al Nizwani, Zoya Shaikh, Asem Shalaby, and Yahyah Tamimi The FASEB Journal 2019 33:1_supplement, lb135-lb135

18 Zolkipli-Cunningham Z, Falk MJ. Clinical effects of chemical exposures on mitochondrial function. Toxicology. 2017; 391:90-99. doi: 10.1016/j.tox.2017.07.009

19 Bruce Lipton, The Biology of Belief, Fall 2009. (San Francisco State University: SFSU Speaker Archives. http://www.sfsu.edu/~holistic/Welcome.html (accessed 08/21/20012).

20 https://en.wikipedia.org/wiki/Psychoneuroimmunology

21 Seeman, T., Dubin, L. and Seeman, M. (2003). Religiosity/spirituality and health: A critical review of the evidence for biological pathways. American Psychologist, 58, 53-63.

22 Lancaster K, Goldbeck L, Puglia MH, Morris JP, Connelly JJ. DNA methylation of OXTR is associated with parasympathetic nervous system activity and amygdala morphology. Soc Cogn Affect Neurosci. 2018;13(11):1155-1162. doi:10.1093/scan/nsy086

23 Ryan Jones; 'Brain Battery'; December 14, 2012; https://knowingneurons.com/2012/12/14/brain-battery/

24 https://www.brucelipton.com/blog/what-are-the-volts-electricity-your-human-body

25 Essentials of Anatomy & Physiology. "Voltage-Gated Channels and the Action Potential." The McGraw-Hill Co., Video. 2016.; http://highered.mheducation.com/sites/0072943696/student_view0/chapter8/animation__voltage-gated_channels_and_the_action_potential__quiz_1_.html.

26 Nelson, David L, and Michael M Cox. 2013. Lehninger Principles of Biochemistry 6th Ed. Book. 6th ed. New York: W.H. Freeman and Co. doi: 10.1016/j.jse.2011.03.016.

27 P. Michael Conn, "Cell Polarity in Development and Disease": A volume in Perspectives in Translational Cell Biology; 2017; https://doi.org/10.1016/C2014-0-02606-8

28 Camfferman, D. (1999) Energy Medicine: The New Health Frontier and the Coming Millennium. Alive, 196, 10-11.

29 Oschman JL, Chevalier G, Brown R. The effects of grounding (earthing) on inflammation, the immune response, wound healing, and prevention and treatment of chronic inflammatory and autoimmune diseases. J Inflamm Res. 2015; 8:83-96. Published 2015 Mar 24. doi:10.2147/JIR.S69656

30 Chevalier G, Sinatra ST, Oschman JL, Delany RM. Earthing (grounding) the human body reduces blood viscosity-a major factor in cardiovascular disease. J Altern Complement Med. 2013;19(2):102-110. doi:10.1089/acm.2011.0820

31 Ghaly M. Teplitz D. The biological effects of grounding the human body during sleep, as measured by cortisol levels and subjective reporting of sleep, pain, and stress. J Altern Complement Med. 2004;10:767–776.

32 Davidson VL. Sittman DB. Biochemistry, 3rd ed. The National Medical Series for Independent Study. Philadelphia, Baltimore, Hong Kong, London, Munich, Sydney & Tokyo: Harwal Publishing; 1994.

33 Oschman JL. Can electrons act as antioxidants? A review and commentary. J Altern Complement Med. 2007;13:955–967.

34 Sokal K, Sokal P. Earthing the human body influences physiologic processes. J Altern Complement Med. 2011;17(4):301-308. doi:10.1089/acm.2010.0687

35 www.ultimatelongevity.com/earthing-grounding/products/index.shtml

36 Atakan Z. (2012). Cannabis, a complex plant: Different compounds and different effects on individuals. DOI:10.1177/2045125312457586

37 Cannabidiol (CBD): Pre-review report. (2017).who.int/medicines/access/controlled substances/5.2_CBD.pdf

38 ElSohly MA, et al. (2016). Changes in cannabis potency over the last 2 decades (1995–2014): Analysis of current data in the United States. DOI:10.1016/j.biopsych.2016.01.004

39 https://cbdhealthwellness.info/2019/09/13/everything-you-need-to-know-about-the-endocannabinoid-system/ extracted November 28, 2020

40 https://www.healthline.com/health/endocannabinoid-system#how-it-works/ extracted November 28, 2020

41 Ahn K, et al. (2008). Enzymatic pathways that regulate endocannabinoid signaling in the nervous system. DOI:1021/cr0782067

42 Gomez M, et al. (2008). Cannabinoid signaling system.ncbi.nlm.nih.gov/pmc/articles/PMC2633685

43 Russo EB. Clinical Endocannabinoid Deficiency Reconsidered: Current Research Supports the Theory in Migraine, Fibromyalgia, Irritable Bowel, and Other Treatment-Resistant Syndromes. Cannabis Cannabinoid Res. 2016;1(1):154-165. Published 2016 Jul 1. doi:10.1089/can.2016.0009

44 https://simplinano.com/blogs/news/a-simple-guide-to-the-endocannabinoid-system/ extracted November 28, 2020

45 Trappe, T. et al (2006) Cardiorespiratory responses to physical work during and following 17 days of bed rest and spaceflight. Journal of Applied Physiology; 100: 951–957.

46 Axillary dissection versus no axillary dissection in patients with sentinel-node micrometastases (IBCSG 23-01): a phase 3 randomised controlled trial. Galimberti V, et.al.; International Breast Cancer Study Group Trial 23-01 investigators.; Lancet Oncol. 2013 Apr;14(4):297-305. doi: 10.1016/S1470-2045(13)70035-4. Epub 2013 Mar 11., PMID: 23491275

47 https://www.britannica.com/science/effector-cell, extracted October 31,2020

48 https://en.wikipedia.org/wiki/Immunological_memory

49 Ingham, B. and Smialowska, A. and Kirby, N. M. and Wang, C. and Carr, A. J., A structural comparison of casein micelles in cow{,} goat and sheep milk using X-ray scattering. Soft Matter. 2018,v14, ISS17,3336-3343, The Royal Society of Chemistry, doi 10.1039/C8SM00458G,http://dx.doi.org/10.1039/C8SM00458G

50 Lv S, Wang Q, Zhao W, et al. A review of the postoperative lymphatic leakage. Oncotarget. 2017;8(40):69062-69075. Published 2017 Apr 20. doi:10.18632/oncotarget.17297

51 https://www.cancer.org/cancer/cancer-causes/antiperspirants-and-breast-cancer-risk.html

52 Caffo M, Caruso G, Fata GL, et al. Heavy metals, and epigenetic alterations in brain tumors. Curr Genomics. 2014;15(6):457-463. doi:10.2174/1389202915066150106151847

53 Miska-Schramm A, Kapusta J, Kruczek M. The Effect of Aluminum Exposure on Reproductive Ability in the Bank Vole (Myodes glareolus). Biol Trace Elem Res. 2017;177(1):97-106. doi:10.1007/s12011-016-0848-3

54 Jessen NA, Munk AS, Lundgaard I, Nedergaard M. The Glymphatic System: A Beginner's Guide. Neurochem Res. 2015;40(12):2583-2599. doi:10.1007/s11064-015-1581-6

55 Phylameana lila Desy;" What is Hilot?"; May 19. 2019: https://www.learnreligions.com/what-is-hilot-1729136

56 Nicolas Dutzan, Loreto Abusleme, Hayley Bridgema, Yasmine Belkai, Joanne E. Konkel, Niki M. Moutsopoulos; On-going Mechanical Damage from Mastication Drives Homeostatic Th17 Cell Responses at the Oral Barrier, Open Access Published: January 10, 2017, DOI:https://doi.org/10.1016/j.immuni.2016.12.010

57 Society for General Microbiology. (2010, September 6). Talented bacteria make food poisoning unpredictable. ScienceDaily. Retrieved June 19, 2020 from www.sciencedaily.com/releases/2010/09/100905231235.htm

58 Warburg OH. On the origin of cancer cells. Science. 1956; 123:309–21. doi: 10.1126/science.123.3191.309

59 Tennant SM, Hartland EL, Phumoonna T, et al. Influence of gastric acid on susceptibility to infection with ingested bacterial pathogens. Infect Immun. 2008;76(2):639-645. doi:10.1128/IAI.01138-07

60 Graham DY, Smith JL, Patterson DJ. Why do apparently healthy people use antacid tablets? Am J Gastroenterol. 1983;78(5):257-260.

61 https://www.drugtopics.com/community-practice/antacid-sales-top -10-billion-annually

62 Andrea Cattaneo, Nicola Tecce, Marco Derudi, Simone Gelosa, Giuseppe Nano & Domenico Maria Cavallo (2014) Assessment of Modeled Indoor Air Concentrations of Particulate Matter, Gaseous Pollutants, and Volatile Organic Compounds Emitted from Candles, Human and Ecological Risk Assessment: An International Journal, 20:4, 962-979, DOI: 10.1080/10807039.2013.821902

63 Knight, L., A. Levin, AND C. Mendenhall. Candles and Incense as Potential Sources of Indoor Air Pollution: Market Analysis and Literature Review (EPA/600/R-01/001). U.S. Environmental Protection Agency, Washington, D.C., 2001.

64 Knight, L., A. Levin, AND C. Mendenhall. Candles and Incense As Potential Sources Of Indoor Air Pollution: Market Analysis And Literature Review (EPA/600/R-01/001). U.S. Environmental Protection Agency, Washington, D.C., 2001.

65 Nriagu JO, Kim MJ. Emissions of lead and zinc from candles with metal-core wicks. Sci Total Environ. 2000;250(1-3):37-41. doi:10.1016/s0048-9697(00)00359-4

66 de Kok, Theo & Hogervorst, Janneke & Kleinjans, Jos & Briedé, Jacob. (2005). Radicals in the church. The European respiratory journal: official journal of the European Society for Clinical Respiratory Physiology. 24. 1069-70. 10.1183/09031936.04.00113404.

67 Stephan Weber, Exposure of Churchgoers to Airborne Particles; Environmental Science & Technology 2006 40 (17), 5251-5256; DOI: 10.1021/es0517116

68 Kotecha AM, Corrêa ADC, Fisher KM, Rushworth JV. Olfactory Dysfunction as a Global Biomarker for Sniffing out Alzheimer's Disease: A Meta-Analysis. Biosensors (Basel). 2018;8(2):41. Published 2018 Apr 13. doi:10.3390/bios8020041

69 https://www.mayoclinic.org/diseases-conditions/gastroparesis/ symptoms-causes, extracted October 31, 2020

70 https://medlineplus.gov/ency/anatomyvideos/000097.htm, extracted November 29, 2020

71 https://medlineplus.gov/ency/anatomyvideos/000097.htm, extracted November 29, 2020

72 "Practical Dietetics With Special Reference To Diet In Disease", by William Gilman Thompson, MD, PhD

73 Sun WM, Houghton LA, Read NW, Grundy DG, Johnson AG. Effect of meal temperature on gastric emptying of liquids in man. Gut. 1988;29(3):302-305. doi:10.1136/gut.29.3.302

74 Longo, V. D. & Mattson, M. P. Cell Metab. 19, 181–192 (2014)

75 Litterbach EV, Campbell KJ, Spence AC. Family meals with young children: an online study of family mealtime characteristics, among Australian families with children aged six months to six years. BMC Public Health. 2017;17(1):111. Published 2017 Jan 24. doi:10.1186/s12889-016-3960-6

76 Michael Pollan, In Defense of Food: An Eater's Manifesto. New York: Penguin Press. 2008.

77 Rickman JC, Bruhn CM and Barrett DM, Nutritional comparison of fresh, frozen, and canned fruits and vegetables. Part 2. Vitamin A and carotenoids, vitamin E, minerals and fibre.J Sci Food Agric in press

78 https://www.biodynamics.com/biodynamic-principles-and-practices

79 Łuszczki E, Sobek G, Bartosiewicz A, et al. Analysis of Fruit and Vegetable Consumption by Children in School Canteens Depending on Selected Sociodemographic Factors. Medicina (Kaunas). 2019;55(7):397. Published 2019 Jul 22. doi:10.3390/medicina55070397

80 Anantha Lakkakula, et.al. Repeated taste exposure increases liking for vegetables by low-income elementary school children, Appetite,Volume 55, Issue 2,2010,Pages 226-231,ISSN 01956663,https://doi.org/10.1016/j.appet.2010.06.003.

81 Bass J. Circadian topology of metabolism. Nature. 2012; 491:348–356.

82 Van Cauter E., Polonsky K.S., Scheen A.J. Roles of circadian rhythmicity and sleep in human glucose regulation. Endocr. Rev. 1997; 18:716–738.

83 Galgano, Fernanda & Favati, Fabio & Caruso, Marisa & Pietrafesa, A & Natella, Stefano. (2007). The Influence of Processing and Preservation on the Retention of Health-Promoting

Compounds in Broccoli. Journal of food science. 72. S130-5. 10.1111/j.1750-3841.2006.00258.x.

84 Joy Yang, 'The Human Microbiome Project: Extending the definition of what constitutes a human', July 16. 2012; https://www.genome.gov/27549400/the-human-microbiome-project-extending-the-definition-of-what-constitutes-a-human

85 Wehrens SMT, Christou S, Isherwood C, et al. Meal Timing Regulates the Human Circadian System. Curr Biol. 2017;27(12):1768-1775.e3. doi:10.1016/j.cub.2017.04.059

86 David Oliver, "Microbes and You: Normal Flora," The Science Creative Quarterly, August 2003

87 Staley JT, Reysenbach AL, eds. 2002. Biodiversity of Microbial Life: Foundation of Earth's Biosphere. New York: Wiley. 552p.

88 English MP. 1982. Microbes, Man, and Animals: The Natural History of Microbial Interactions. New York: Wiley. 342p.

89 Jenness R. The composition of human milk. Semin Perinatol. 1979 Jul;3(3) 225-239. PMID: 392766.

90 Joy Yang, "The Human Microbiome Project: Extending the definition of what constitutes a human," July 16. 2012; https://www.genome.gov/27549400/the-human-microbiome-project-extending-the-definition-of-what-constitutes-a-human

91 https://www.genome.gov/27549400/the-human-microbiome-project-extending-the-definition-of-what-constitutes-a-human

92 Zeeuwen, P et al. Microbiome dynamics of human epidermis following skin barrier disruption. Genome Biology 2012; 13: R101.

93 https://www.dermnetnz.org/topics/microorganisms-found-on-the-skin

94 Bell V, Ferrão J, Pimentel L, Pintado M, Fernandes T. One Health, Fermented Foods, and Gut Microbiota. Foods. 2018;7(12):195. Published 2018 Dec 3. doi:10.3390/foods7120195

95 Sender R, Fuchs S, Milo R. Revised Estimates for the Number of Human and Bacteria Cells in the Body. PLoS Biol. 2016;14(8):e1002533. Published 2016 Aug 19. doi: 10.1371/journal.pbio.1002533

96 Kiela PR, Ghishan FK. Physiology of Intestinal Absorption and Secretion. Best Pract Res Clin Gastroenterol. 2016;30(2):145-159. doi: 10.1016/j.bpg.2016.02.007

97 Vitetta L, Chen J, Clarke S. The vermiform appendix: an immunological organ sustaining a microbiome inoculum. Clin Sci (Lond). 2019;133(1):1-8. Published 2019 Jan 3. doi:10.1042/CS20180956

98 Wu SC, Chen WT, Muo CH, Ke TW, Fang CW, Sung FC. Association between appendectomy and subsequent colorectal cancer development: an Asian population study. PLoS One. 2015;10(2):e0118411. Published 2015 Feb 24. doi:10.1371/journal.pone.0118411

99 Canton G, Santonastaso P, Fraccon IG. Life events, abnormal illness behavior, and appendectomy. Gen Hosp Psychiatry. 1984;6(3):191-195. doi:10.1016/0163-8343(84)90039-2

100 Enblad M, Birgisson H, Ekbom A, Sandin F, Graf W. Increased incidence of bowel cancer after non-surgical treatment of appendicitis. Eur J Surg Oncol. 2017;43(11):2067-2075. doi:10.1016/j.ejso.2017.08.016

101 Hempel S, Newberry SJ, Maher AR, et al. Probiotics for the prevention and treatment of antibiotic-associated diarrhea: a systematic review and meta-analysis. JAMA. 2012;307(18):1959-1969. doi:10.1001/jama.2012.3507

102 Butel MJ. Probiotics, gut microbiota, and health. Med Mal Infect. 2014;44(1):1-8. doi: 10.1016/j.medmal.2013.10.002

103 Guarner F, Khan AG, Garisch J, et al. World Gastroenterology Organisation Global Guidelines: probiotics and prebiotics October 2011. J Clin Gastroenterol. 2012;46(6):468-481. doi:10.1097/MCG.0b013e3182549092

104 Zhernakova, Alexandra et.al., Population-based metagenomics analysis reveals markers for gut microbiome composition and diversity},352,6285, 565—569,2016, 10.1126/science. aad3369, American Association for the Advancement of Science

105 Bell V, Ferrão J, Pimentel L, Pintado M, Fernandes T. One Health, Fermented Foods, and Gut Microbiota. Foods. 2018;7(12):195. Published 2018 Dec 3. doi:10.3390/foods7120195

106 A.C. Ouwehand, H. Röytiö, 1 - Probiotic fermented foods and health promotion, Editor(s): Wilhelm Holzapfel, In Woodhead Publishing Series in Food Science, Technology and Nutrition, Advances in Fermented Foods and Beverages, Woodhead

Publishing, 2015, Pages 3-22, ISBN 9781782420156, https://doi.org/10.1016/B978-1-78242-015-6.00001-3.

107 R.F. Mcfeeters, Fermentation Microorganisms and Flavor Changes in Fermented Foods, Vol. 69, Nr. 1, 2004—Journal of Food Science, https://fbns.ncsu.edu/USDAARS/Acrobatpubs/P322-328/P325.pdf

108 G. Mena-Sánchez, et.al., Fermented dairy products, diet quality, and cardio–metabolic profile of a Mediterranean cohort at high cardiovascular risk, Nutrition, Metabolism and Cardiovascular Diseases, Volume 28, Issue 10, 2018, Pages 1002-1011, ISSN 0939-4753, https://doi.org/10.1016/j.numecd.2018.05.006.

109 Ramírez-Garza SL, Laveriano-Santos EP, Marhuenda-Muñoz M, et al. Health Effects of Resveratrol: Results from Human Intervention Trials. Nutrients. 2018;10(12):1892. Published 2018 Dec 3. doi:10.3390/nu10121892

110 Kechagia M, Basoulis D, Konstantopoulou S, et al. Health benefits of probiotics: a review. ISRN Nutr. 2013; 2013:481651. Published 2013 Jan 2. doi:10.5402/2013/481651

111 Delhanty PJD, van der Lely AJ (eds): How Gut and Brain Control Metabolism. Front Horm Res. Basel, Karger, 2014, vol 42, pp 83-92. doi: 10.1159/000358316

112 Ruth Ann Luna, Jane A Foster, Gut brain axis: diet microbiota interactions and implications for modulation of anxiety and depression, Current Opinion in Biotechnology, Volume 32,2015, Pages 35-41, ISSN 0958-1669, https://doi.org/10.1016/j.copbio.2014.10.007.

113 Suparna Roy Sarkar, Sugato Banerjee, Gut microbiota in neurodegenerative disorders, Journal of Neuroimmunology, Volume 328,2019, Pages 98-104, ISSN 0165-5728, https://doi.org/10.1016/j.jneuroim.2019.01.004.

114 Kang JH, Yun SI, Park MH, Park JH, Jeong SY, Park HO. Anti-obesity effect of Lactobacillus gasseri BNR17 in high-sucrose diet-induced obese mice. PLoS One. 2013;8(1):e54617. doi: 10.1371/journal.pone.0054617

115 Alshami AM. Pain: Is It All in the Brain or the Heart? Curr Pain Headache Rep. 2019 Nov 14;23(12):88. doi: 10.1007/s11916-019-0827-4. PMID: 31728781.

116 Martinucci I, Blandizzi C, de Bortoli N, et al. Genetics and pharmacogenetics of aminergic transmitter pathways in functional gastrointestinal disorders. Pharmacogenomics. 2015;16(5):523-539. doi:10.2217/pgs.15.12

117 Advances in Enteric Neurobiology: The "Brain" in the Gut in Health and Disease - Scientific Figure on ResearchGate. Available from: https://www.researchgate.net/figure/Organization-of-the-enteric-nervous-system-within-the-gut-wall-of-the-small-intestine_fig1_328644662 [accessed 29 Nov, 2020]

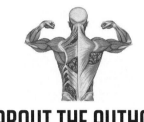

ABOUT THE AUTHOR

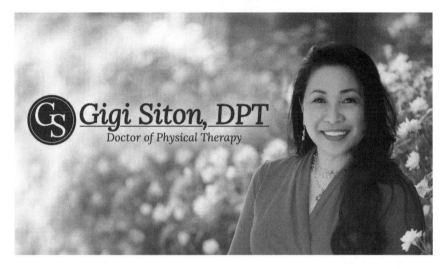

Dr. Gigi Siton, DPT
www.gigisiton.com

Dr. Gigi Siton, DPT, founder, and CEO of Holistic Physical Therapy, has a doctorate in physical therapy with almost thirty years of clinical experience. She is the author of multiple books: (1) *"THE SEXY ART OF HIGH-HEEL WALKING": How To Wear High Heels Pain-free*; (2) *"YOUR BODY IS A SELF-HEALING MACHINE"* Trilogy - *"Your Body Is A Self- Healing Machine"* Trilogy - Book 1: *"Understanding Epigenetics – Why It Is Important To Know"*; Book 2: *"Understanding the Anatomy of Epigenetics"*; Book 3: *"Understanding How Epigenetics Heals You."* She was one of the speakers at the Personal Improvement Symposium, Harvard University Faculty Club, on

September 20 & 12, 2017. For almost eight years at her Holistic Physical Therapy Clinic, she has taught a monthly class called *"Nutritional Bootcamp: A Practical Class on Epigenetics 101."*

She finished her Doctorate in Physical Therapy from Simmons College, Boston, MA, and a Bachelor of Science in Physical Therapy from De La Salle University, Cavite, Philippines. She also has a Bachelor of Science in Psychology from the University of Santo Tomas, Manila, Philippines. She is also a Nutritional Therapy Practitioner (NTP).

She has worked in inpatient acute care, neuro, stroke, spinal cord injuries, post-surgical orthopedic rehabilitation in inpatient and outpatient settings, labor and delivery, neonatal babies, inpatient and outpatient pediatrics, and wound and burn care, school setting, cardiac rehab acute, and outpatient. For the past seventeen years, she has worked in an outpatient physical therapy setting for acute and chronic pain management, pelvic floor rehab, orthopedic rehab, vertigo rehab, sports medicine, and nutritional medicine.

In 2013, she finally opened her own Holistic Physical Therapy Clinic north of Houston. It is a holistic practice that addresses the root cause of the problem, not just the symptoms. She believes that this holistic physical therapy approach is the cornerstone of any comprehensive and holistic health program. The six keys to holistic health and healing are: nutritional, physical, emotional, social, environmental, and spiritual. When your body works the way that nature intended, your spirit soars—and therefore, so do you.

Her physical therapy style is a combination of Eastern philosophy with Western medicine training and sensibilities. She has further enhanced her skills with years of training in traditional physical therapy interventions combined with additional advanced training in a myofascial trigger point release, acupuncture, internal Qigong, yoga, Pilates on mat and the reformer, whole-body vibration therapy, energy medicine, manual manipulation, visceral manipulation, kinesiotaping, and TRX with sports medicine.

Texas Monthly Magazine named her Five-Star Physical Therapist two years in a row and a recipient of the 2015 Houston Medical Awards for Best Physical Therapy Clinic.

In 1989, she was directly hired to work for Conroe Regional Hospital as a Licensed Physical Therapist in an acute care setting. She came from very humble beginnings. She is the tenth child of twelve children from the southern island of the Philippines called Mindanao. She has eight sisters and three brothers. Oroquieta City is her beloved hometown, where all her passion and inner core started. Her father was a criminal lawyer, state prosecutor, and dean of the College of Law. He was brutally assassinated on August 29, 1985. Her mother was also an educator with a master's in elementary education. She died in her sleep from a broken heart two and a half years after her father's passing. With God's blessing, all her siblings have finished college and post-graduate studies. They all have successful careers.

She is a single mother who loves spending time with her two daughters, Ally and Victoria. She is an eternal student, a voracious reader, loves to dance and travel. She loves meeting people and making them smile and helping them feel better about themselves.

Her mission in life: *"I intend to make people feel better about themselves because they met me."*

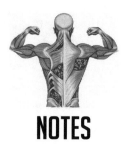

NOTES

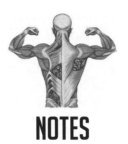

NOTES

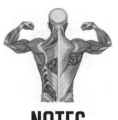

NOTES